THE LIES WE EAT:

Beginners Guide to Decoding Food Labels for Understanding to Make Healthier Dietary Choices

Introduction

Reading labels, why is it important?

Chemicals can be found everywhere, in everything. Everything is a chemical because everything is made of matter. What is matter? Matter is anything that has mass and volume or takes up space. The question is not whether what you are consuming is a chemical or contains chemicals. The question is whether the chemicals in the product are harmful or dangerous.

The word chemical is not a "bad" word. Afterall, we cannot live without dihydrogen monoxide right!? Of course not. Being comprised of anywhere from 60-74% water, people will die without it. Therefore, it is important to be well informed and educated, the goal of this e-book. By the end of this read, if one person is left feeling more confident about reading a label and making an informed decision for themselves and their family, then this was not in vain.

As a formally trained chemist and a mom, I am an avid label reader. When I started, 15 years ago, there was not nearly as much information readily available to support self-education and training as there is today.

In the beginning, I toiled for hours in the grocery aisles as I learned more about what I was feeding my kids and trying to find suitable substitutes. It was a struggle and while I was not able to eliminate all added sugars and all artificial ingredients, I have been able to make some positive changes while still allowing my kids to enjoy many of their favorite snacks and foods. My children are not vegetarian nor vegan. Neither am I. Moderation is our mantra in life.

The iconic Nutrition Facts label was introduced more than 20 years ago to help consumers make informed food choices and maintain healthy dietary practices. There is so much information that it is easy to become overloaded. The do's and do not's of nutrition is ever changing. The purpose of this read is to compile and present the best information currently available in a way that is easy to read, understand, and apply. Education is the goal.

Chapter 1: The Label

What is on a label? Food labeling is required for most prepared foods. Lots of useful information can be gained by reading food labels, including its origin, the ingredients, whether the food is organic, natural, or genetically modified. Additionally, types of nutrients and any health claims are also found there. This information can be use to help you make healthy food choices.

The Food Label Includes the Following Parts:

1. Food Product Name: This will include the brand and common name of the product and may also include a picture.
2. Net Contents: This information represents the entire weight, including fluid content, the amount listed is in common household amounts (pounds/ounces) and metric measures (grams/milliliters).
3. Manufacturer's Name and Address: This information is provided so that you can contact the company should you have any questions or concerns regarding the product.

Nutrition Facts Label

On the nutrition facts label, manufacturers are required to provide information on certain nutrients. The mandatory nutrients are total calories, calories from fat, total fat, saturated fat, trans fat, cholesterol, sodium, total carbohydrates, dietary fiber, sugars, protein, vitamin A, vitamin C, calcium, and iron. If a claim is made about any other ingredient or nutrient, the manufacturer is required to include that information.

A food label must also include a list of Ingredients in decreasing order by weight. This list is required on all foods with more than one ingredient.

Nutrient Content Claims

Words and phrases that may be use to describe the amount of a nutrient in a food but does not tell exactly how much. Some nutrient content claims that may be seen on a food product label include: "Low Fat," "Sugar-Free," "Fat-Free," "Low-Calorie," or "Reduce Sodium.

Health Claims

Describe how a food or food component such as fat, calcium, iron, or fiber relates to a disease or health-related condition.   Only health claims supported by scientific evidence are allowed on labels. Currently, there are eight health claims that have been approved. They include:

1. Calcium and osteoporosis;
2. Fat and cancer;
3. Saturated fat,
4. cholesterol and heart disease;
5. Fiber containing grain products;
6. fruits, vegetables and cancer;
7. Fruits, vegetables and grain products that contain fiber and heart disease;
8. Sodium and high blood pressure;
9. Folic acid and neural tube birth defects.

Product Date

There are two types of product dating. They are Open Dating and Code Dating. Open Dating is stamped on a product package to help the store determine how long to display the product for sale. This date can also help you to know when to buy or use the product for best flavor and quality. There are four types of open dating:

1. "Sell by" - This is the last day the product should be sold or used by the store. Usually, this date allows for additional storage and use time at home.

2. "Best if Used By (Before)" - Use the product by this date for the best flavor and quality. This is not a food safety date.
3. "Expiration Date" or "Use by" - This is the last day the product should be used or eaten.
4. "Pack Date" - This is the date when the food was packaged or processed.

Code Dating is used on foods that can be stored on the shelf for a longer time, such as canned or packaged foods. This date is used by manufacturers.

Importance of label reading

Reading food labels will make it much easier for you to compare data and find the foods that have the nutritional value you and your family need. This can aid in making healthy choices about the foods you are buying.

Food labels also tell exactly what is inside the package. Just look at the list of Ingredients. The first ingredient represents the ingredient with the most amount, the second ingredient is the second highest amount and so on.

Food is not simple anymore. It exists mostly in multiples and variations. There is a plethora of options for rice, mind-boggling assortments of grains and a deluge of edible oils available for today's foodie. In such a scenario, it is natural to shop extra, and shop mindlessly. If a major portion of your diet is coming out of a box, bag, or a can, you should definitely be aware of what your truly consuming. Therefore, not only is reading food labels important, it is imperative.

Food labels can help you limit the amount of fat, sugar and cholesterol in your diet by making it easy for you to compare one food item with another and choose the one with lower amounts. Conversely, you can use food labels to find food items higher in vitamins, fiber and protein.

One essential detail that is commonly overlooked is that the nutritional information found on a food label is based on <u>one-serving</u> of that particular food. This is one of the most common mistakes people make when reading food labels. A food label may indicate that a food has 100 calories and only 5 grams of sugar, for example. But if you look at the number of servings, it may state three. That means that if you were to eat the entire package, you would be getting three times the amount shown on the food label. In this example, 300 calories and 15 grams of sugar. Do not be fooled! Always look at what makes one-serving. Remember this is what the food label information is based on. Additionally, know how many servings are in that package. It is important to note that some serving sizes have changed on the new Nutrition Facts label, according to the Food and Drug Administration's website. By law, serving sizes must be based on the amount of food people typically consume, rather than how much they should consume. Serving sizes have been updated to reflect the amount people typically eat and drink today. For example, based on the review of relevant information such as nationwide surveys of the amounts of foods Americans eat, the serving size for soda has changed from 8 ounces to 12 ounces. Additionally, the Food and Drug Administration (FDA) allows a company to label a food as "fat-free" if it contains less than 0.5 grams of fat per serving. There is so much more to label reading and food labeling. This is just the tip of the iceberg.

The Point

Food labels tell you about the contents, serving size, number of servings in the package, calories per serving and the amount of various nutrients present in the product. As an educated buyer you can compare the labels to determine which foods are lowest in calories, fat, saturated fat, trans fat, cholesterol, sodium and sugar, and pick the least unhealthy item. Today many foods are preserved, flavored, blended, texturized, thickened, and colored with FDA approved additives, but even when labels state "all natural" or "USDA approved," harmful chemicals may still be present. Therefore, understanding labels is vital to choosing the right packaged foods.

All ready-made foods come with a nutrition label describing what you are consuming. Understanding each of those ingredients helps you make healthier choices. Checking food labels also makes it easy for you to compare the nutrient content of different options. It helps you avoid certain Ingredients if you have a food intolerance or are following a diet that excludes certain components, such as dairy or gluten.

Chapter 2: The History of the American Diet

The Federal government has provided dietary advice for the public for more than 100 years through bulletins, posters, brochures, books, and—more recently—websites and social media. Dietary guidance has generally included advice about what to eat and drink for better health, but the specific messaging has changed throughout the years to reflect advances in nutrition science and the role of specific foods and nutrients on health.

The earliest focus of dietary guidance was on food groups in a healthy diet, food safety, food storage, and ensuring that people get enough minerals and vitamins to prevent certain diseases that occur when a vitamin or mineral is lacking. As nutrition science evolved, there was greater recognition of how the diet can play a role in disease prevention and health promotion. In 1980, the first publication of the Dietary Guidelines for Americans was released. Since then, these guidelines have become the cornerstone of Federal food and nutrition guidance.

Senate Select Committee on Nutrition and Human Needs

A turning point for nutrition guidance in the U.S. began in the 1970s with the formation of the Senate Select Committee on Nutrition and Human Needs. This Committee came into existence as a bridge between interests in the Senate Agriculture Committee and the Labor and Public Welfare Committee. In its early years, the Senate Committee focused on programs designed to eliminate hunger, but more evidence linking diet to the "Nation's killer diseases" was building. This allowed the Senate Committee to expand its focus and investigate how nutrition related to the overall health of Americans. The Senate Committee indicated that:

- Healthy diets could play an important role in promoting health, increasing productivity, and reducing health care costs.
- The American diet has changed within the last 50 years, and people need guidance to improve their health through better nutrition.
- The government has a role to provide nutrition guidance to Americans and encourage the advancement of nutrition research and industry food reformulation.

In 1977, after years of discussion, scientific review, and debate, the U.S. Senate Select Committee on Nutrition and Human Needs, led by Senator George McGovern, released Dietary Goals for the United States. The Dietary Goals recommended:

- To avoid being overweight, consume only as much energy as is expended.
- If overweight, decrease energy intake and increase energy expenditure.
- Increase the consumption of complex carbohydrates and "naturally occurring" sugars from about 28 percent of intake to about 48 percent of energy intake.
- Reduce the consumption of refined and processed sugars by about 45 percent to account for about 10 percent of total energy intake.
- Reduce overall fat consumption from approximately 40 percent to about 30 percent of energy intake.
- Reduce saturated fat consumption to account for about 10 percent of total energy intake; and balance that with polyunsaturated and monounsaturated fats, which should account for about 10 percent of energy intake each.
- Reduce cholesterol consumption to about 300 milligrams a day.
- Limit the intake of sodium by reducing the intake of salt to about 5 grams a day.

- Changes in food selection and preparation to help individuals with achieving the Dietary Goals were also suggested.

Following the release of the Dietary Goals, some groups and individuals expressed doubt that the science available at the time supported the specificity of the recommendations. To support the credibility of the science use by the Senate Committee, the U.S. Department of Agriculture and an organization called Health and Human Services or HHS (then called the Department of Health, Education, and Welfare), selected scientists from the two departments and obtained additional expertise from the scientific community throughout the country to address the public's need for authoritative and consistent guidance on diet and health.

USDA and HHS Collaborate to develop the Dietary Guidelines

In February 1980, the USDA and HHS collaborated and issued the Nutrition and Your Health: Dietary Guidelines for Americans, which described seven principles for a healthful diet to help healthy people in making daily food choices. This edition was based, in part, on the 1979 Surgeon General's Report on Health Promotion and Disease Prevention and the findings from a task force convened by the American Society for Clinical Nutrition, which reviewed the evidence relating six dietary factors to the Nation's health. The focus of the 1980 Dietary Guidelines was to offer ideas for incorporating a variety of foods in the diet to provide essential nutrients while maintaining recommended body weight.

This edition also provided guidance on limiting dietary components such as sugar, bad fat like saturated and trans-fat, and sodium, which were beginning to be seen as risk factors in certain chronic diseases. Both the Dietary Goals and the first Dietary Guidelines for Americans were different from previous guidance in that they reflected evolving scientific evidence and changed the historical focus on nutrient adequacy to also identify the impacts of diet on chronic disease. These guidance documents discussed the concepts of moderation, including alcohol consumption, as well as nutrient adequacy.

Similar to the Dietary Goals, the 1980 Dietary Guidelines was met with controversy from some groups and individuals. This led to the use of an external Advisory Committee.

Utilizing a Federal Advisory Committee to Review the Science

After the release of the 1980 Dietary Guidelines, Congress directed the USDA and HHS to convene a Federal advisory committee to seek outside scientific expert advice prior to the Departments developing the next edition of guidelines. Thus, a Dietary Guidelines Advisory Committee was established, composed of scientific experts entirely outside the Federal sector, The advisory committee's scientific report helped to inform the development of the 1985 Nutrition and Your Health: Dietary Guidelines for Americans. While relatively few changes from the 1980 edition were made, this second edition was issued with much less debate. These guidelines were used as the framework for consumer nutrition education messages. They also were used as a guide for healthy diets by scientific, consumer, and industry groups.

In 1989, USDA and HHS established a second scientific advisory committee to review the 1985 Dietary Guidelines and make recommendations for the next revision. The guidance of the earlier release was reaffirmed. The 1990 Nutrition and Your Health: Dietary Guidelines for Americans promoted enjoyable and healthful eating through variety and moderation, rather than dietary restriction.

USDA and HHS have continued to charter a Dietary Guidelines Advisory Committee for each subsequent revision cycle. Each committee is tasked with reviewing the science on nutrition and health, receiving and reviewing public comments, and preparing scientific reports to advise the government. These scientific reports informed the USDA and HHS as the departments developed the 1995, 2000, 2005, 2010, 2015-2020, and 2020-2025 editions of the Dietary Guidelines.

Evolving Focus: From Nutrients to Dietary Patterns

Since 1980, the Dietary Guidelines have been notably consistent on what components make up a healthy diet, but they also have evolved in some significant ways to reflect updates to the science.

Previous editions of the Dietary Guidelines relied on the body of science looking at the relationships between individual nutrients, foods, and food groups and health outcomes. Although this science base continues to be substantial, science has progressed. There is now a body of science looking at the relationship between overall dietary patterns and various health outcomes.

Just as nutrients are not consumed in isolation, foods and beverages are not consumed separately either. Rather, consumption occurs in various combinations over time—an eating or dietary pattern. The current science base shows that components of an dietary pattern can have interactive, synergistic, and potentially cumulative relationships, such that the pattern may be more predictive of overall health status and disease risk than individual foods or nutrients. Thus, dietary patterns, and their food and nutrient components, are at the core of the current guidelines for Americans, 2020-2025. This edition of the Dietary Guidelines also takes a lifespan approach focusing on what to eat and drink at different life stages, and confirms the core elements of a healthy eating pattern.

Chapter 3: The Hows of Label Reading

Labels are designed so that consumers are provided with useful information about the product and how this would fit into their daily diets. This is how one could read these labels.

Look at the list of Ingredients

This list provides an overview of the product's "recipe" or constituents. Ingredients are arranged from the maximum to the least amount. E.g.: If a product lists its ingredients as: Sugar, Water, and Juice Concentrate Artificial Flavor-This means that the bulk of the product is sugar. The ingredient with least amount is juice concentrate.

Be aware of health sensitive ingredients

Health-sensitive ingredients include fat, sugar, and salt. The rule for these is "Less is better". Frequent high intake of these ingredients is associated with obesity, heart problems diabetes etc.

Watch the nutrient amounts

The Nutrition Information Label for nutrient amounts are given either per 100 grams of the product or by the recommended Energy and Nutrient Intake amount. This allows you to compare nutrient amounts among different brands of a particular food.

Get more value

Check the real cost per serving of a product and how many servings could be prepared from a large pack. For this, you will need to look at these three things:

1. The net weight. This is the amount of product inside the pack. This can be found near the bottom of a pack, usually at the front of the packaging.
2. The serving size. This is the amount (usually in grams or milliliters) per serving of a product.
3. The price.

Divide Net Weight by Serving Size. This will give you the number of servings in the pack. Next take the number of servings and divide by the price. This will give you the cost per serving and help you decide if the pack is worth the price being charged. If this sounds too complicated, try dividing the total weight of the package by the cost. If you do this for each item comparing, this will give you the cost per unit measure or weight.

Choose low energy-dense foods

Opt for low energy-dense foods. These are foods that contain a higher water content such as soups, stews, pasta dishes, and rices. Energy density refers to the ratio of calories to the weight of the food. Less calories per portion size is generally better for weight management. Eating low energy-dense food will help you feel full due to relatively bigger portion size, yet low caloric amount.

Understanding nutrient content claims

1. A zero-calorie product can actually contain up to 4 calories per serving
2. A fat-free product can contain up to 0.5 grams of fat per serving
3. A low-fat product can have as much as 3 grams for solid products and 1.5g for liquid products.

The Food Label is designed to inform the consumer and aid in making healthy food choices. By knowing how to use it, you can understand how a specific food item can fit into your overall diet. You can more effectively and efficiently select foods and choose between products. So, go ahead, check the label and better manage your health.

Chapter 4: Toxic Ingredients to Avoid

There are thousands of ingredients used to make foods. Consumers demand and enjoy foods that are flavorful, convenient, colorful, affordable, and hopefully nutritious and safe. Food additives and advances in technology help make that possible. The FDA maintains a list of over 3000 ingredients. According to the governing body's website, "FDA can never be absolutely certain of the absence of any risk from the use of any substance. Therefore, FDA must determine - based on the best science available - if there is a reasonable certainty of no harm to consumers when an additive is used as proposed." Over the years, there has been growing concerns about the safety of many common food additives, if consumed in large quantities. While, in many cases, there may be no definitive data linking disease to food additives, here is some food for thought:

Nitrates/Nitrites

Commonly seen on food packaging as sodium nitrate/sodium nitrite, these components are used in processed meats to inhibit bacterial growth. While nitrate itself is harmless; it is readily converted to nitrite. When nitrites combine with compounds called secondary amines, they form nitrosamines: extremely powerful cancer-causing chemicals. The chemical reaction occurs most readily at the high temperatures of frying. Nitrite has long been suspected as being a cause of stomach cancer.

High Fructose Corn Syrup

High fructose corn syrup is a leading cause of obesity and has been fingered as a causative factor in heart disease. It raises blood levels of cholesterol and triglycerides. It makes blood cells more prone to clotting, and it may also accelerate the aging process.

Monosodium glutamate or MSG

MSG is a flavor enhancer and a contributor to obesity. The FDA has classified it as a food ingredient that's "generally recognized as safe." MSG is an excitotoxin, which causes nerve damage and allergic reactions. It is linked to several disorders including reproductive abnormalities, Alzheimer's, brain tumors, as well as dementia to name a few. Found in thousands of foods/prepared products, MSG has many acceptable alternative trade names, making it a challenge to identify. According to a study published in January 2018 in the EXCLI Journal, even the lowest dose of MSG has toxic effects.

Note, some foods contain a natural form of MSG. It is important to understand the body metabolizes, or processes, naturally occurring ingredients differently. It recognizes the pieces and parts of the natural molecule and breaks them down in a way that does not yield the same harmful effects as it would when processing its artificial twin. Thus, the notion regarding the body not being able to tell the difference between artificial substances and natural substances is not all together true.

Sodium Benzoate

Sodium Benzoate, an organic compound, can increase the risk of cancer, specifically leukemia, as well as anemia. Inhalation of high levels can cause headaches, rapid heart rate, tremors, confusion, unconsciousness and death. Exposure can also cause reproductive issues in both men and women alike. Commonly use in detergents, drugs, pesticides and adhesives. It is also used as a preservative, often found in soft drinks.

Benzene, a carcinogen, may form at exceedingly small levels in some carbonated soft drinks that contain both benzoate salts and ascorbic acid. The FDA has no standard for benzene in beverages other than bottled water. For bottled water, the allowable limit is 5 billion (ppb) for drinking water.

Between November 2005 and May 2007, the FDA found that 10 beverage samples contained benzene levels over 5 ppb. All 10 products have either been reformulated or discontinued by their manufacturers. Benzene levels in the reformulated products, if detected at all, were less than 1.5 ppb.

The FDA has determined that that the levels of benzene found in beverages to date do not pose a safety concern for consumers.

BHA/BHT

BHA (butylated hydroxyanisole) and BHT (butylated hydroxytoluene) are closely related synthetic antioxidants used as preservatives in lipsticks and moisturizers, among other cosmetics. They are also widely used as food preservatives, commonly found in some of your favorite cereals.

Banned in other countries, these two preservatives are considered carcinogenic but remain in U.S. manufactured foods that contain oil as they retard rancidity or possessing an unpleasant odor or flavor.

Acrylamide

Acrylamide, a chemical used for thickening, is considered to "likely to be carcinogenic to humans" according to the US Environmental Protection Agency. In laboratory studies, acrylamide caused cancer in animals, but at acrylamide levels much higher than those seen in foods. Acrylamide is a chemical that can form in some foods during high-temperature cooking, such as frying, roasting, and baking, with frying causing the highest formation amount.

Parabens

The most common parabens found in consumer products are methylparaben, propylparaben, ethyl paraben, and butylparaben. Since making their debut in the 1920's, parabens are a group of chemicals widely used as artificial preservatives in cosmetic and body care products. Cosmetics contain ingredients that can biodegrade. As a result, parabens are added to prevent and reduce the growth of harmful bacteria and mold thus increasing the shelf life of the product. The concern with these potentially harmful chemicals is that scientific studies suggest parabens penetrate the skin and act like a very weak estrogen, potentially turning on the growth of hormone-receptor-positive breast cancers. In addition to disrupting hormones in the body, these chemicals can harm fertility and reproductive organs, affect birth outcomes, and increase the risk of cancer. Parabens have been found in breast tissue and breast cancer cells.

Chapter 5: Artificial Sweeteners

When it comes to sugar intake, the American Heart Association recommends that women should have no more than six teaspoons (25 grams) and men should have no more than nine teaspoons (37 grams) of added sugar per day.

Non-nutritive sweeteners or sugar substitutes are sweeteners that are used instead of regular table sugar (sucrose), with artificial sweeteners being one type. The topic of sugar substitutes can be confusing. One problem is that the terminology is often open to interpretation.

These substitutes are considered high-intensity sweeteners because they are many times sweeter than sugar but contribute only a few to no calories when added to foods. Some manufacturers call their sweeteners "natural" even though they are processed or refined. Stevia is one of the best examples. It is derived from naturally occurring substances, as is sucralose. It comes from sugar.

Artificial Sweeteners

If you are trying to reduce the sugar and calories in your diet, you may be turning to artificial sweeteners or other sugar substitutes. You are not alone.

Artificial sweeteners and other sugar substitutes are found in a variety of food and beverages marketed as "sugar-free" or "diet," including soft drinks and baked goods. Just what are all these sweeteners? And what is their role in your diet?

Artificial sweeteners are synthetic sugar substitutes. But they may be derived from naturally occurring substances, such as herbs or sugar itself. Artificial sweeteners are also known as intense sweeteners because they are many times sweeter than sugar.

They can be attractive alternatives to sugar because they add virtually no calories to your diet. Also, you need only a fraction of them compared with the amount of sugar you would normally use for sweetness.

Uses

Artificial sweeteners are widely use in processed foods, including:
- Soft drinks, powdered drink mixes and other beverages
- Baked goods
- Candy
- Puddings
- Canned foods
- Jams and jellies
- Dairy products

They are also popular for home use. Some can even be used in baking or cooking. Certain recipes may need modification because unlike sugar, artificial sweeteners provide no bulk or volume. Check the labels for appropriate home use.

Possible health benefits

Artificial sweeteners do not contribute to tooth decay and cavities. Artificial sweeteners may also help with:
- Weight control. They contain virtually no calories. In contrast, a teaspoon of sugar has about 16 calories — so a can of sweetened cola with 10 teaspoons of added sugar has about 160 calories. If you are trying to lose weight or prevent weight gain, products sweetened with artificial sweeteners may be an attractive option, although their effectiveness for long-term weight loss is not clear.
- Diabetes. Artificial sweeteners aren't carbohydrates. So unlike sugar, they generally do not raise blood sugar levels. Ask your doctor or dietitian before using any sugar substitutes if you have diabetes.

Possible health concerns

Artificial sweeteners have been scrutinized intensely for decades. Critics say that they cause a variety of health problems, including cancer. That is largely because of studies dating to the 1970s that linked the artificial sweetener saccharin to bladder cancer in laboratory rats. Because of those studies, saccharin once carried a label warning that it may be hazardous to your health.

Artificial sweeteners are regulated by the FDA as food additives. They must be reviewed and approved by the FDA before being made available for sale. Sometimes the FDA declares a substance "generally recognized as safe" also referred to as GRAS. Substances receive this designation if they meet either of these criteria:

- Qualified professionals deem the substance safe for its intended use on the basis of scientific data. Stevia preparations are an example of this type of GRAS designation.
- The substances have such a lengthy history of common use in food that they are considered generally safe.

The FDA has established an acceptable daily intake for each artificial sweetener. This is the maximum amount considered safe to consume each day over the course of a lifetime and are set at very conservative levels.

Saccharin

Saccharin, approved for use in food as a non-nutritive sweetener, is 200 to 700 times sweeter than sucrose and does not contain any calories.

First discovered and used in 1879, saccharin is one of the oldest no-calorie sweeteners. In the early 1970s, saccharin was linked with the development of bladder cancer in laboratory rats, which led Congress to mandate additional studies of saccharin and the presence of a warning label on saccharin-containing products until such warning could be shown to be unnecessary. Today, saccharin is currently approved for use without warning or restriction.

Aspartame

Aspartame is approved for use in food as a nutritive sweetener and does contain calories, but because it is about 200 times sweeter than table sugar, consumers are likely to use much less of it.

The FDA approved aspartame in 1981 for uses, under certain conditions, as a tabletop sweetener and in 1966 as a "general purpose sweetener." It is not heat stable and loses its sweetness when heated, so it typically is not used in baked goods. Aspartame is one of the most exhaustively studied substances in the human food supply, with more than 100 studies supporting its safety. FDA scientists have reviewed this data and have concluded that it is safe for the general population under certain conditions. However, people with a rare hereditary disease known as phenylketonuria (PKU) have a difficult time metabolizing phenylalanine, a component of aspartame.

Sucralose

Sucralose is a no-calorie sweetener that contributes sweetness to foods and beverages without adding calories or carbohydrates. It is made from a process that begins with regular sucrose; however, sucralose is not sugar. Most consumed sucralose is not absorbed. Of the small amount absorbed none is broken down for energy, so sucralose does not provide any calories. All absorbed sucralose is excreted quickly in the urine.

The FDA approved its use in specific food categories in 1998 and expanded the approval to all food and beverage categories in 1999.

Natural sweeteners

Natural sweeteners are sugar substitutes that are often promoted as healthier options than sugar or other sugar substitutes. But even these "natural sweeteners" often undergo processing and refining.

Natural sweeteners that the FDA recognizes as generally safe include:
- Fruit juices and nectars
- Honey
- Molasses
- Maple syrup

Allulose, a monosaccharide also known as psicose, is a rare sugar. It is found naturally in dried fruits like jackfruit, figs and raisins, but only in small quantities which makes it difficult to extract from its original source. Allulose is about 70% as sweet as sucrose and is similar in taste. Gram for gram, allulose has approximately 90% fewer calories than sucrose. Allulose is versatile for use in food products that are baked, frozen or in liquid items. It is not metabolized by the body but is instead absorbed by the small intestine and excreted in the urine. Because of this, allulose does not increase blood glucose or insulin levels.

Uses
Natural sweeteners have a variety of uses both at home and in processed foods. They are sometimes known as "added sugars" because they are added to foods during processing.

Possible health benefits
Natural sugar substitutes may seem healthier than sugar despite their vitamin and mineral content having little if any significant difference. For example, honey and sugar are nutritionally similar, and your body processes both into glucose and fructose. It is OK to choose a natural sweetener based on how it tastes rather than on its health claims. A good rule of thumb is to use any added sweetener sparingly.

Possible health concerns
Natural sweeteners are generally safe however there is no health advantage to consuming any type of added sugar. Consuming too much added sugar, even natural sweeteners, can lead to health problems, such as tooth decay, weight gain, poor nutrition and increased triglycerides. Honey can contain

small amounts of bacterial spores that can produce botulism toxin. Honey should not be given to children younger than one year old.

Novel sweeteners

Novel sweeteners are hard to fit into a particular category because of what they are made from and how they are made. They are typically a combination of different types of sweeteners. Basically, this is the category for sweeteners that do not fall into any of the above categories.

Tagatose

Tagatose is also considered a novel sweetener because of its chemical structure. Tagatose is a sugar like fructose. It is a low carbohydrate sweetener that occurs naturally but is manufactured from the lactose in dairy products, specifically whey. The FDA categorizes tagatose as a GRAS substance.

Stevia

A well-known sweetener, Stevia, is the most well-known example of a novel sweetener. Grown naturally in tropical climates, stevia is an herb in the chrysanthemum family that grows wild as a small shrub in Paraguay and Brazil, though it can easily be cultivated elsewhere. Paraguayans have used stevia as a food sweetener for centuries while other countries, including Brazil, Korea, Japan, China and much of South America, have a shorter, though still long-standing, record of stevia use.

Sugar alcohols

Sugar alcohols, or polyols, are carbohydrates that occur naturally in certain fruits and vegetables — although they can also be manufactured. Despite their name, sugar alcohols aren't alcoholic because they do not contain ethanol, which is found in alcoholic beverages.

Polyols aren't considered intense sweeteners because they aren't sweeter than sugar. In fact, some are less sweet than sugar. As with artificial sweeteners, the FDA regulates the use of them. They contain calories but are lower in calories than sugar, making them an attractive alternative.

Uses
Polyols generally are not used when preparing food at home. But they are in many processed foods and other products, including chocolate, chewing gum and toothpaste. Sugar alcohols add sweetness, bulk and texture to food, as well as helping food to stay moist.
Polyols are often combined with artificial sweeteners to enhance sweetness. Food labels may use the general term "sugar alcohol" or list the specific name, such as sorbitol and maltitol.

Possible health benefits
Polyols are not metabolized by oral bacteria, and so they do not contribute to tooth decay. They do contribute calories to your diet — but fewer calories than regular sugar. As a result, polyols may help weight-control efforts.

Unlike artificial sweeteners, these sweeteners are carbohydrates and can raise blood sugar levels. But your body does not completely absorb sugar alcohols, so their effect on blood sugar is smaller than that of other sugars.

Possible health concerns
In the body, sugar alcohols travel to the large intestine where they are metabolized by gut bacteria. These bacteria then release hydrogen gas. As a result, eating too many foods sweetened with sugar alcohols over a short period of time can cause gas, bloating and stomach pain. When eaten in large amounts, sugar alcohols can have a laxative effect, causing bloating, intestinal gas and diarrhea. Product labels may carry a warning about this potential laxative effect.

Moderation is key

When choosing sugar substitutes, it pays to be a savvy consumer. Artificial sweeteners and sugar substitutes can help with weight management. But they are not a magic fix for choosing sweet flavor over proper health and nourishment. Like everything in life, use should be in moderation.

Food marketed as sugar-free is not calorie-free, so it can still cause weight gain. Keep in mind that processed foods, which often contain sugar substitutes, generally do not offer the same health benefits as whole foods, such as fruits and vegetables.

Chapter 6: Processed Foods

The term "processed food" can cause some confusion because most foods are processed in some way. Mechanical processing — such as grinding beef, heating vegetables, or pasteurizing foods — does not necessarily make foods unhealthful. If the processing does not add harmful chemicals or ingredients, it does not tend to lessen the healthfulness of the food.

However, there is a difference between mechanical processing and chemical processing. Chemically processed foods often only contain refined ingredients and artificial substances, with little nutritional value. They tend to have added chemical flavoring agents, colors, and sweeteners. These ultra-processed foods are sometimes called "cosmetic" foods, as compared with whole foods. Some examples of ultra-processed foods include:

- frozen or ready meals
- baked goods, including pizza, cakes, and pastries
- packaged breads
- processed cheese products
- breakfast cereals
- crackers and chips
- candy and ice cream
- instant noodles and soups
- reconstituted meats, such as sausages, nuggets, fish fingers, and processed ham
- sodas and other sweetened drinks

Are processed foods bad for you?

Ultra-processed foods tend to taste good and are often inexpensive. These foods are food and drink products that have undergone specified types of food processing, usually by transnational and other exceptionally large 'Big food' corporations. However, they usually contain Ingredients that could be harmful if consumed in excess, such as saturated fats, added sugar, and salt. These foods also contain less dietary fiber and fewer vitamins than whole foods.

One large study, involving more than 100,000 adults, found that eating 10% more ultra-processed foods was associated with above a 10% increase in the risks of cardiovascular disease, coronary heart disease, and cerebrovascular disorders. This conclusion was reached after accounting for saturated fat, sodium, sugar, and fiber intake.

Another large study, involving almost 20,000 adults, found that eating more than 4 servings of processed food daily was linked with an increased risk of all-cause mortality, or death from any cause. For each additional serving, all-cause mortality risk increased by 18%.

While the research links ultra-processed foods to several health problems, it also shows that people tend to eat more of these foods leading to an increase rate of obesity. Additionally, it takes the body much longer to digest these foods due to their high-fat content. As a result, they tend to cause more belly fat. One recent study even tied the convenience foods to cancer risk.

Below, we look at seven reasons why processed foods can increase the risk to a person's health.

Added sugar

Processed foods tend to contain added sugar and, often, high fructose corn syrup. Added sugar contains no essential nutrients but is high in calories. Regularly consuming an excess of added sugar can lead to compulsive overeating. It is also linked with health conditions such as obesity, metabolic syndrome, type 2 diabetes, and inflammatory diseases.

Processed foods and beverages are among the major sources of added sugar in the diet. Sweetened beverages are a particularly significant source as people tend to consume much more sugar than they realize in soft drinks. Cutting down on added sugar — by drinking sparkling water instead of soda, for example — is a quick and effective way to make the diet more healthful.

Artificial Ingredients

The ingredients list on the back of processed food packaging is often full of unrecognizable substances. Some are artificial chemicals that the manufacturer has added to make the food more palatable.

Highly processed foods often contain the following types of chemicals:

preservatives
Food preservatives enhance the life span of foodstuffs, which suggests that food spoilage is well protected. It results in reduced wastage and enhanced supply. Preservatives can cause allergic reactions especially in people with asthma. They have been linked to cancer. Sodium nitrate and sodium nitrite are used to preserve meat and have been found to produce cancer-causing chemicals called nitrosamines. Preservatives are also harmful to children. Food additives can negatively impact and interfere with a child's hormones, growth, and development, potentially causing consequences as wide-ranging as infertility, obesity, cardiovascular disease, and decreased immunity.

artificial coloring
The first artificial food colorings were created in 1856 from coal tar. Nowadays, food dyes are made from petroleum. Over the years, hundreds of artificial food dyes have been developed, but most have since been found to be toxic. There are only a handful of artificial dyes that are still used in food. Food manufacturers often prefer artificial food dyes over natural food colorings, such as beta carotene and beet extract, because they produce a more vibrant color. However, there is quite a bit of controversy regarding the safety of artificial food dyes. Not everyone agrees with that conclusion. Interestingly, some food dyes are deemed safe in one country, but banned from human consumption in another, making it extremely confusing to assess their safety.

chemical flavoring
Of the three chemical senses, smell is the main determinant of a food item's flavor. Both natural and artificial flavors are synthesized in

laboratories, but artificial flavors come from petroleum and other inedible substances, while "natural flavor" must be derived from plant or animal material. A great deal of scientific engineering and design time goes into crafting flavors for processed foods.

texturing agents
Food Texturing agents are food additives which are chemical substances, used to change the texture or "mouthfeel" of the food by providing it with the characteristics such as creaminess and thickness. They also play a key role in increasing shelf life of the product by giving it a stable structure.

Processed foods can contain dozens of additional chemicals that are not listed on their labels.   For example, "artificial flavor" is a proprietary blend. Manufacturers do not have to disclose exactly what it means, and it is usually a combination of potentially harmful chemicals. While most food additives have been tested for "safety," the use of these chemicals remains controversial among doctors and researchers.

Refined carbohydrates

Carbohydrates are an essential component of any diet. However, carbs from whole foods provide far greater health benefits than refined carbohydrates.

Highly processed foods are often high in refined carbs. The body breaks down refined, or simple, carbohydrates quickly, leading to rapid spikes in blood sugar and insulin levels, thus consuming them is linked with an increased risk of type 2 diabetes. With frequent changes in blood sugar and insulin levels, a person may experience food cravings and low energy.

Healthy sources of carbohydrates include:
- oats, barley, or bran.
- whole-grain bread.
- brown rice.
- plenty of fresh fruit and vegetables.
- fresh, whole fruit instead of juice.

- whole-grain pasta.
- salads and raw vegetables.

Low in nutrients

Ultra-processed foods are extremely low in essential nutrients, compared with whole or minimally processed foods. In some cases, manufacturers add synthetic vitamins and minerals to replace nutrients lost during processing. However, whole foods provide additional healthful compounds that ultra-processed foods do not.

Fruits, vegetables, and grains, for example, contain healthful plant compounds with antioxidant, anti-inflammatory, and anticarcinogenic effects. These include flavonoids, anthocyanins, tannins, and carotenoids. The best way to get the full range of essential nutrients is to eat whole, unprocessed, or minimally processed foods.

Low in fiber

Dietary fiber has a wide range of health benefits. Fiber can slow the absorption of carbohydrates and help people feel more satisfied with fewer calories. It also acts as a prebiotic, feeding the friendly bacteria in the gut, and can help boost heart health.

Most ultra-processed foods are incredibly low in fiber, as natural fiber is lost during processing. Healthful high fiber foods include:

- Pears
- Strawberries
- Avocado
- Apples
- Raspberries
- Bananas
- Carrots
- Beets
- Broccoli
- Artichoke

- Brussel sprouts
- Lentils
- Kidney beans
- Split peas
- Chickpeas
- Quinoa
- Oats
- Popcorn
- Almonds
- Chia seeds
- Sweet potatoes
- Dark chocolate

If you find yourself consuming greater than acceptable quantities of processed or ultra-processed foods, snacking on the above list of high fiber foods may help offset any undesirable effects.

Quick calories

The way that manufacturers process foods makes them very easy to chew and swallow. Because much of the fiber is lost during processing, it takes less energy to eat and digest ultra-processed foods than whole or less processed foods. As a result, it is easier to eat more of these products in shorter periods. In doing so, a person consumes more calories — and uses fewer in digestion — than they would if they had eaten whole foods instead. This increases a person's chances of taking in more calories than they use, which can lead to unintentional weight gain.

Trans fats

Ultra-processed foods are often high in unhealthy cheap fats. For example, they often contain refined seed or vegetable oils, which can be easy to use, inexpensive, and last a long time. Manufacturers create artificial trans fats by adding hydrogen to liquid vegetable oils, making them more solid. Trans fats increase inflammation in the body. They also raise levels of low-density lipoprotein, or "bad," cholesterol, and decrease levels of high-density lipoprotein, or "good," cholesterol.

Eating trans fats is associated with an increased risk of heart disease, stroke, and type 2 diabetes. For example, according to a 2019 study, a 2% increase in energy intake from trans fats is linked with a 23% increase in cardiovascular risk. The best way to avoid refined oils and trans fats is to avoid processed foods. One can replace these with healthy alternatives, such as avocado, flaxseed, or olive oils.

Chapter 7: The Dirty Dozen

Buying organic carries a higher price tag than conventional produce, but there are ways you can reduce the cost by growing your own produce, joining a co-op, or getting organic vegetable boxes delivered to your door.

If you are buying produce conventionally, there are two especially important lists to be familiar with; they are the clean 15 and the dirty dozen. These lists provide some guidance on where focus and emphasis at the marketplace should be honed when making cost effective decisions. In these lists, you will find a break down of what produce has the least and most amount of pesticides and is a great place to start when choosing what is crucial to purchase organic, and what is passable as non-organic.

Have a read below to find out more about what organic means and read through the clean 15 and dirty dozen list for your next shopping trip.

What is organic food?

According to the Organic Foods Production Act, the definition of an organic product is "animal products sold or labeled as organically produced, are not given any kind of antibiotics or growth hormones, are only fed with organic feed, and are not administered any type of medication aside from vaccinations or to treat illness." Fruits and vegetables that are labeled and sold as organic are grown without using most pesticides or fertilizers with synthetic ingredients. There is no irradiation treatment, seeds and transplants are chemical-free, and the fertilizer is natural.

USDA National Organic Program NOP sets the regulations in the organic industry. Products labeled as "100% organic" must contain only organically produced ingredients and processing aids, excluding water and salt. No other ingredients or additives are permitted. Products labeled "organic" must contain at least 95% organically produced ingredients (excluding water and salt). Any remaining ingredients must consist of non-agricultural substances that appear on the NOP National List of Allowed and Prohibited Substances.

What are the health benefits of organic food?

For starters, better nutrition. A study found that organic fruits and veggies contain 27% more vitamin C, 21.1% more iron, 29.3% more magnesium, 13.6% more phosphorus, and 18% more polyphenols than non organic produce. While being higher in these nutrients, they are also significantly lower in nitrates and pesticide residues. The function of pesticides is to act as a selective poison. Food that is grown with the use of pesticides and herbicides carry this potential risk to the consumer. Buying organic lowers this risk.

Dirty Dozen List for 2020

This list was comprised by the Environmental Working Group and is listed in order of the most contaminated fruits and vegetables.

1. Strawberries
2. Spinach
3. Kale
4. Nectarines
5. Apples
6. Grapes
7. Peaches
8. Cherries
9. Pears
10. Tomatoes
11. Celery
12. Potatoes

Chapter 8: Balanced Diet?

A good diet is important for our health and can help us feel our best but what is a good diet? Apart from breastmilk as a food for babies, no single food contains all the essential nutrients the body needs to stay healthy and work properly. For this reason, our diets should contain a variety of different foods, to help us get the wide range of nutrients that our bodies need.

A balanced diet is not a fad, yo-yo or crash diet. It is a way of ensuring you eat all of the required nutrients for your body to function properly. A balanced diet will not be the same for everyone. Overall nutritional needs are essentially the same though each of us have varying nutritional requirements based on body type, genetic predisposition, age, gender, and activity levels. Thus, each of us require different amounts and types of nutrients. What you need will depend on age, gender, lifestyle, health and the rate at which your biological systems function.

Eating a balanced diet is key in maintaining good health and keeping your body in optimum condition. A balanced diet does not cut out food groups; it consists of a wide variety of foods to support your body and keep you energized, motivated and healthy.

It may sound simple, but with so much information available, messages about "healthy eating" can become unclear. Facts become fads and knowing what is good for you can be misunderstood. The following are some general guidelines on foods necessary to support healthy dietary balance and support staying hydrated as well as information about how a nutrition professional can support you.

How much food do I need to have a healthy diet?
A healthy diet should provide the right amount of energy (calories or kilojoules), from foods and drinks to maintain energy balance. Energy balance is where the calories taken in from the food sources are equal to the calories use by the body in the form of energy, preferably work. We need these calories to carry out every day tasks

such as walking and moving about, but also for all the functions of the body we may not even think about. Processes like breathing, pumping blood around the body and thinking also require calories.

Foods and drinks provide the calories we need to go about our daily lives, but consuming more calories than we need over a period can, and in most cases does, cause weight gain. This is because, any extra calories consumed and not used will just be stored as fat.

According to the research, nearly 40% of American adults aged 20 and over are obese. 71.6% of adults aged 20 and over are overweight, including obesity. (*National Health and Nutrition Examination Survey*, 2017-2018; *Harvard School of Public Health*, 2020). Based on CDC reports, the prevalence of obesity from 2015 to 2016, for children and adolescents aged 2-19 years, was 18.5%. Obesity prevalence was 13.9% among 2- to 5-year-olds, 18.4% among 6- to 11-year-olds, and 20.6% among 12- to 19-year-olds. Being overweight as a child increases the risk of developing type 2 diabetes, heart disease and some cancers in adulthood. So, maintaining a healthy weight is really important for health.

How much energy you need from foods and drinks depends on many different things, such as how active you are. But on average:

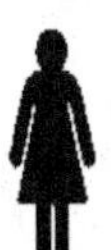

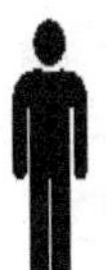

Eating only as many calories as you need will help to maintain a healthy weight. However, the foods and drinks you choose need to be the right ones, and in the right proportions to stay healthy.

Whether you're just starting your wellness journey or you are a professional athlete, speaking to a nutrition professional can be greatly beneficial. It is easy to get wrapped up in what you see and hear in the media, but what works for one person may not be right for you. If you have a goal, whether it be as simple as getting healthier and looking after your body or running a marathon, there will be certain foods your body needs. Speaking to a professional can help you identify any changes you can make to help you reach your goal.

The journey can be lonely, especially if those close to you do not understand what you're doing. A nutrition professional can provide the support you need, push you out of your comfort zone and keep you motivated, all the while educating you on your body and what a balanced diet means to you.

You may be required to complete a food diary before your session, as well as answer some questions to help the professional get a clear understanding of where any issues may lie. If you have any questions, ask. It is important for the professional to know what's on your mind, so they know how to help. Together, you will be able to create a personalized diet plan, tailored to your needs, depending on your goal, your lifestyle or your health concern.

Chapter 9: Portion sizes

Carbohydrates and starchy foods, such as rice, pasta, cereal and potatoes, should generally be the size of your fist. Butter and spreads are often high in fat and sugar, therefore only a small amount is needed - aim for a portion the size of the tip of your thumb. Protein sources, such as meat and fish, should generally be the size of your palm.

Fruit and vegetables will generally make up the largest part of your meals. Try to add a variety of greens to your lunch and dinners and if you can snack on fruit, you can easily reach the 5 a day recommendation.

Once again, portion sizes will vary. If you exercise regularly, you may need more food than someone who is not very active - in this case, a sports nutritionist may be able to help you.

Reference intakes

Reference intakes or recommended daily amounts are used as general guidelines to determine what the average person needs. These can be found on the back of food and drink packaging and can help us understand what is in foods. Similar to the traffic light system printed on the front of most food packaging, knowing what we are eating can encourage us to make healthier choices.

5 a day: Fruits & Veggies

The 5 a Day program in the United States was originally the National Fruit and Vegetable Program but was rebranded as Fruits & Veggies – More Matters. Fruits & Veggies – More Matters is a national public health initiative from Produce for Better Health Foundation and the CDC to better communicate updated dietary guidelines, which recommended more than 5 servings of fruits and vegetables for some Americans.

The processes in our bodies, such as the digestive system, the circulatory system, and the immune system, all require certain minerals to function. Fortunately, there are many fruits and vegetables available, all ranging in shape, size, taste and nutritional value.

Copper, iron, potassium and zinc are four minerals that are essential to the body. While vitamins A, B6 and vitamin C are key in our growth and providing us with energy. To learn more about which minerals and vitamins are found in which foods, and how they can benefit your health, please contact a nutrition professional.

One way to up your intake of vegetables is to reduce your meat intake and enjoy more vegetarian meals. A plant-focused diet has been linked to a reduced risk of cancer and other chronic diseases and may play a role in maintaining a healthy gut microbiome, which can affect the risk of chronic disease and obesity.

Saturated and unsaturated fat

There are two types of fat that can be found in food, saturated and unsaturated. Unsaturated fat can help lower cholesterol and provide essential fatty acid, omega-3. Found in oily fish, such as mackerel, tuna and salmon, avocado, nuts, and olive oil, unsaturated fat can also help the body absorb vital vitamins, such as vitamin A, D and E.

Saturated fat can be found in cakes, biscuits, crisps, hard cheese and pastry. Eating an excess of saturated fat can lead to health problems as it can raise cholesterol in the blood which, in turn, increases the risk of developing heart disease.

Protein

Protein is essential for the body and helps develop and repair muscles. We can find this in meat, fish, beans, eggs, diary and tofu. Protein seems to have gained popularity and while it is beneficial to the body, too much can be detrimental. If you are concerned about your protein intake and want to know more, contact a nutrition professional.

Salt

Salt is naturally present at low levels in all foods but around 80% of our salt intake is hidden in processed food. Most of the salt children and adults eat is hidden in processed and convenience foods, and the rest comes from salt added during cooking and any salt added at the table.

According to the American Heart Association, Our Salty Six infographic shows the top six sodium sources in the U.S. diet.

These include:
1. Breads and Rolls
2. Pizza
3. Sandwiches
4. Cold Cuts and Cured Meats
5. Soup
6. Burritos and Tacos

Staying Hydrated

What does it mean to be hydrated? The amount of water a person needs depends on climatic conditions, clothing worn, and exercise intensity and duration. Someone who perspires heavily will need to drink more than someone who does not. Certain medical conditions, such as diabetes or heart disease, may also mean you need to drink more water. People with cystic fibrosis have high concentrations of sodium in their sweat and need to use caution to avoid dehydration. Some medications can act as diuretics, causing the body to lose more fluid requiring increased hydration efforts as well.

We all need water to survive. However, there is more to drinking water than being properly hydrated. Water acts as our body's solvent. It carries waste, nutrients and other important components around our body, as well as keeping our skin and hair healthy. Outdated literature suggest aiming for around six to eight eight-ounce glasses. In more recent data, the suggestion is to drink between half an ounce and an ounce of water for each pound you weigh, every day. For me, being approximated 150 pounds my water intake daily should be 75 ounces to 150 ounces. Ultimately, proper hydration can be best indicated by the color of your urine and should be monitored. Dark colored urine suggests your kidneys are conserving water due to dehydration, where as pale-yellow urine indicates a well-hydrated body.

Sugars and starchy foods

There are two types of sugar - refined and unrefined. It is naturally found in many foods, including fruits, vegetables, dairy, grains, and even nuts and seeds. This natural sugar can be extracted to produce the refined sugar currently so abundant in the food supply. Table sugar and high-fructose corn syrup are two common examples of refined sugars created this way. Table sugar, or sucrose, is typically extracted from sugar cane plants or sugar beets.

The sugar manufacturing process begins with washing the sugar cane or beets, slicing them, and soaking them in hot water, which allows their sugary juice to be extracted.

The juice is then filtered and turned into a syrup that is further processed into sugar crystals that are washed, dried, cooled, and packaged into the table sugar. Refined sugars are added to food, for example in sweets, desserts, and fizzy drinks. Too much refined sugar can be harmful to the body. Refined sugar intake is linked to conditions like obesity, type 2 diabetes, and heart disease.

Unrefined sugars contain mainly sucrose, but also glucose and fructose — as opposed to white sugar, which is made up of almost pure sucrose. They generally have over 90% total sugars, being 88–95% sucrose, and 2–7% invert sugar (glucose plus fructose). Unrefined sugar in moderation can be beneficial for the body and provides a quick, effective burst of energy.

Starchy foods are often the victim of many crash diets, with people 'cutting carbs' in an attempt to lose weight. However, starchy foods play a vital role in maintaining a balanced diet. Starchy foods such as grains, pulses, oats and bread provide slow-releasing energy, as well as being good sources of fiber, calcium, iron and vitamin B. Whole grain varieties are recommended, as they generally contain more fiber, supporting the digestive system and keeping you fuller for longer.

Meat

Based on a report released in October 2015 by the World Health Organization, processed meat has been classified as carcinogenic to humans. The report states that based on sufficient evidence in humans, the consumption of processed meat causes colorectal cancer, which is any cancer that affects the colon and the rectum. While this association was observed mainly for colorectal cancer, associations were also seen for pancreatic cancer and prostate cancer.

Chapter 10: Sugar, the devil you know

After the Jesuits' introduction of sugar in 1751, sugar became less expensive to produce, thanks in large part to slavery. Sugar consumption has risen steadily ever since.

The following is a history of average sugar consumption per person, per year:

1821: 10 lbs.

1880: 38 lbs.

1970: 119 lbs.

1990: 132 lbs.

2007: 158 lbs.

2017: 170 lbs.

Sugar is contained in many, many foods. Sugar wreaks havoc with many of the body's physiological systems and plays a central role in the current heart disease, cancer, diabetes, and obesity epidemics. Sugar is a super-concentrated, unnatural food. In the past 75 years, our modern industrial culture has seen a unique convergence of many negative lifestyle factors that have lead to a dramatic increase in 'lifestyle behavior diseases' which include heart disease, diabetes, hypertension, obesity, senile dementia, and cancer. This "Perfect Storm" of disease-producing lifestyle behavior choices includes the following:

- A decrease in the intake of micro-nutrients and trace elements within our food supply due to commercial farming practices utilizing year-round growth cycles and nitrogen-based petrochemical fertilizers.
- Creating epidemic nutritional deficiencies or malnutrition within modern industrial nations, as well as food processing methods that strip nearly all nutrients from our food.
- An increase in toxicity of our food supply due to the use of chemical pesticides and herbicides in combination with modern food processing techniques utilizing chemical additives, and preservatives.

- An increase in consumption of food that has been processed to the point where there is little to no nutritive value.
- And a pronounced decrease in physical activity levels unprecedented in the history of mankind.

Refined sugars, or simple carbohydrates, such as sugar, versus sugar cane, or apple juice, versus an apple, have been stripped of their natural fibers. This allows for rapid digestion into the blood stream, which then causes blood glucose levels to spike. This results in over-secretion of insulin, the carrier hormone that transports glucose from the blood to the cells and tissues. Normally, insulin secretion is gradual, corresponding to the gradual absorption of sugars found in complex carbohydrates. When eating refined sugar or corn syrup, the sudden demand for insulin becomes acute and insulin is 'dumped' into the bloodstream. This acute demand for insulin production and secretion overwhelms the pancreas, the organ that produces and secretes insulin. It gets worse: over time, sustained levels of insulin, from continuing to eat refined carbohydrates such as sugar, corn syrup, and white flour – the diet of many Americans, results in insulin resistance, a chronic but deadly condition where the body's cells do not respond to insulin in a normal or healthy manner, causing even more insulin to be secreted. This spike in insulin thus aggravates insulin resistance syndrome even further, creating a self-perpetuating cycle which ultimately leads to many disease processes including atherosclerosis (clogging of the arteries), cancer, diabetes, weight gain/obesity, high blood lipids (abnormal LDL: HDL cholesterol levels), and mineral depletion. Now with an unlimited supply and unlimited access to foods containing sugar or corn syrup, as a society, we are totally hooked. Sugar is without a doubt addictive. Not only is it addictive, but it is also deadly. It destroys your health by leading to obesity and diabetes, causes mineral loss, disrupts hormone function, depress immune system, causing chronic disease, and increase cancer risk.

Sugar Decreases Immune Function

It has long been known that sugar intake causes decreased immune system function. Studies have shown that the immune system is weakened substantially within minutes of eating refined sugar; the more you eat, the more your body's insulin response system is compromised. The body's cell-mediated immunity, which uses specialized white blood cells called neutrophils to attack tumors, viruses and bacteria, is decreased when there is elevated blood glucose, which is caused by eating refined carbohydrate foods such as sugar and white flour.

Sugar and disease (dis-ease)
More research is needed to understand the relationship between sugar in the diet and cancer. All kinds of cells, including cancer cells, depend on blood sugar (glucose) for energy. But giving more sugar to cancer cells does not make them grow faster. The idea that sugar, or glucose, could fuel the growth of cancer cells can lead some people to unnecessarily avoid all carbohydrate containing foods. This approach assumes that if cancer cells need glucose, then cutting it out of one's diet will stop cancer from growing. Unfortunately, it is not that simple. All our healthy cells need glucose to function, and there is no way for our bodies to let healthy cells have the glucose they need, but not give it to the cancer cells. Without adequate carbohydrate intake from foods we eat, our bodies will make glucose from other sources, including protein and fat. Glucose is that critical for our cells to survive and function properly.

Not consuming enough carbohydrates can lead to the breakdown of protein stores in our body, which can contribute to muscle loss and possibly malnutrition. Following a restricted diet with very low amounts of carbohydrates can also cause unintentional weight loss. This can impact the ability to tolerate cancer treatment. Restricting carbohydrates also eliminates foods that are good sources of fiber, vitamins, minerals and immune supporting phytonutrients, a substance found in certain plants which is believed to be beneficial to human health and help prevent various diseases.

To date, there are no randomized controlled trials showing sugar causes cancer. There is, however, an indirect link between sugar and cancer. Eating a lot of high sugar foods such as cakes, cookies, and sweetened beverages can contribute to excess caloric intake. This may lead to weight gain and excess body fat. Research has shown that being overweight or obese increases the risk of 11 types of cancers including colorectal, postmenopausal breast, ovarian, and pancreatic cancer.

While it is not necessary to completely avoid sugar, reducing added sugars and consuming nutrient-dense, high fiber carbohydrates may be most effective.

Current death statistics:

- 1 out of every 4 people will die of heart disease.
- 1out of every 6 people will die from cancer.
- Between 2000 and 2016, there was a 5% increase in premature mortality from diabetes. Obesity is the defining risk factor for heart disease, cancer, and diabetes
- According to CDC statistics (2017-2018):
    - Percent of adults aged 20 and over with obesity: 42.5% Percent of adolescents aged 12-19 years with obesity: 21.2%
    - Percent of children aged 6-11 years with obesity: 20.3%
    - Percent of children aged 2-5 years with obesity: 13.4%

The most startling aspect of these statistics is that all of those diseases were nonexistent, or very rare occurrences, in earlier times amongst the hunter-gatherer cultures that determined the genetic code that our bodies live by today. In other words, the diseases so common today are best described as lifestyle diseases, or behavior diseases.

Addiction

Did you know that in some studies researchers found SUGAR to be more addictive than COCAINE!? This in part is thanks to a feel-good chemical in which our brain produces, DOPAMINE. When you eat something sugary whether it is a cupcake, a candy bar, or even a wholesome piece of fruit, your brain releases a pleasure-giving dopamine response. For most, this satisfies the craving. For many, there is a compulsive desire to repeat that pleasure or "high" when it is too strong to resist. The more sweets you eat, the more required to get that high again. As a result, your body becomes more insulin resistant. This behavior drives our tolerance for sugar higher, thus requiring more sugar.

Addiction is only one part of the problem. Below you will find some of the side effects from the over-consumption of SUGAR, feeding the notion that Sugar is the Devil.

Weight Gain

When your blood glucose levels rise, your body responds by stimulating insulin response as previously mentioned. Again, this is a natural response, triggering your body to flip the on switch to activate fat or energy storing mode. The more consistent you are with your sugar consumption, the longer and more frequently your body will operate in fat storing mode.

If you find yourself on the wrong side of the scale, limit your sugar consumption, and start to research the glycemic index. This system ranks carbohydrates on a scale from 1 to 100 based on their effect on blood sugar levels.

Immune System Suppression

Sugar intake has the ability to suppress your immune system after consumption. According to Health Services at Columbia University, when you eat 100 grams of sugar, about as much sugar as you find in a 1-liter bottle of soda, your white blood cells are 40 percent less effective at killing germs. This can cripple your immune system for up to 5 hours after eating sugar!

Type 2 Diabetes

Type 2 diabetes occurs as a result of a lack of insulin production or an increased resistance to insulin. Insulin is a hormone produced by the pancreas that allows for the regulation of the uptake of glucose (sugar). It is released in response to increased glucose levels in the blood and allows for individual cells to take up glucose from the blood to metabolize it. A high-sugar diet has been linked with an increased incidence of Type 2 diabetes due to the links between high sugar intake and obesity. Over the years excess sugar consumption can cause our bodies to quite possibly stop producing insulin all together. Some complications due to diabetes include blindness, amputation of appendages, depression, neuropathy, sexual dysfunction, kidney disease, and dementia to name a few.

Heart Disease

In numerous studies, a direct link has been shown between increased sugar consumption and death from cardiovascular disease. When insulin levels spike continuously the endothelial lining of the blood vessels become damaged which creates can inflammation. This chronic inflammation, coupled with high blood pressure, excess weight, poor heart health, is what may eventually lead to heart attack.

Inflammation In Your Gut

When your body digests sugar it changes the ratio of good bacteria to bad bacteria in your gut...And not in a good way. Bad bacteria thrives off of sugar and can cause tons of different ailments since they produce all sorts of harmful toxins. Besides feeling run down and low energy, the increase in these toxic bacteria can cause yeast infections, autoimmune disorders, arthritis, heart disease, and many other ailments.

Absorption of Vitamins and Minerals

For most, the consumption of sugar does not yield positive health and fitness benefits. Considering refined sugar lacks significant nutrients, vitamins, or minerals, elimination is the best answer. In fact excess sugar consumption can consequently deplete the body of zinc, magnesium, potassium, and chromium.

Promotes Cancer Cell Growth

In recent studies. sugar is referred to as "fuel" for cancer cells. This may seem extreme, but it is true. As stated earlier, sugar is the fuel for all cells in the body. Sugar is a carbohydrate, and when you eat any type of carbohydrate, refined or unrefined, the pancreas produces insulin, a hormone that helps convert sugars into energy for your cells. Eating too much sugar can cause the body to become insulin resistant, meaning it has to churn out more and more of the hormone in order to do its job.

Adding to much of what has already been mentioned pertaining to sugar and disease, a hormone known as insulin-like growth factor (IGF), which research has shown to stimulate cell growth and inhibit cell death allows cancer to proliferate. Cancer cells are normally kept in check by the body's constant turnover—new healthy cells grow and bad cells die. With an excess of IGF, the signals are blocked that allows for cells to grow normally and die when it is time to die, so instead they just grow and grow and grow.

So next time you are reaching for your sweets, think twice about what you're putting inside your body. Are you prepared to live with the consequences of your actions?

Chapter 11: You are what you eat

Have you ever heard the phrase "You are what you eat?" This phrase is the notion that to be fit and healthy you need to eat good food. In a literal sense, we all can agree that it is true that "you are what you eat." Nutrients from the foods we eat provide the foundation of the structure, function, and wholeness of every cell in our body, from the skin and hair to the muscles, bones, digestive and immune systems. While we may not feel it, we are constantly repairing, healing and rebuilding our body.

Every cell in our body has a "shelf life." A stomach cell lives about a day or two, a skin cell about a month, and a red blood cell about four months. So, every day, our body is busy making new cells to replace those that have "expired." And how healthy those new cells are is directly determined by how well we have been living and ultimately eating. A diet filled with highly processed food that is low in nutrients does not give our body the fuel it needs to be productive and healthy. Alternatively, a clean, nutrient rich, whole foods regimen can help us build cells that work better and are less susceptible to premature aging, inflammation, death, and disease.

There is also strong evidence that, as a rule, the closer to nature you eat, the fewer calories it will take for you to feel satisfied. Why? Processed foods often have low amounts of fiber and water. A lack of fiber can mean an unhealthy digestive system, which can lead to both short and long-term health complications. Low-fiber diets have been linked to dangers like colon cancer, unhealthy cholesterol levels, and diverticulosis. Processed foods also tend to contain a mix of tastes from added sugar, salt, and flavoring that overly stimulate the appetite center in the hypothalamus.

Clean foods are minimally processed and as direct from nature as possible. They are whole and free of additives, colorings, flavorings, sweeteners, and hormones. Some examples include foods with one-word Ingredients like spinach, blueberries, almonds, salmon, and lentils. Clean foods are opposite of processed foods in that they contain lots of fiber and fluid, a high ratio of nutrients to calories, and are free of added flavors. All of these send signals of satisfaction to our brain before we consume excess calories. For example, think of how many raw almonds we eat before stopping in contrast to the honey roasted almonds and that sugary coating. By eating clean, we can control our weight permanently without feeling deprived or hungry or having constant cravings.

Here are the foods you should be eating more of:
- Vegetables
- Fruits
- Nuts and seeds -and-
- Whole grains

And if you are a carnivore, lean sources of protein like fish, duck, ostrich, venison and turkey are great options opposed to chicken, pork, and beef.

The key is to start small. Try eating one or two more servings of vegetables than you normally do this week. Eat a handful of nuts as a snack instead of potato chips. Cook yourself a healthy breakfast, lunch, or dinner instead of going out to eat. Remember, you are what you eat. So, fuel your body with the right foods, and it will reward you for making healthy choices. Healthy food leads to a healthy body, which, in turn, increases your odds of a longer, happier life.

Chapter 12: Trust and The Food Industry

The global food industry has never faced more challenges. From tainted dairy products to contaminated beef, high-profile cases crop up regularly to dent consumer confidence, while leading companies work hard to reclaim lost faith. So, how trustworthy is your food?

Food safety is something we tend to take for granted. When we scan well-stocked supermarket shelves to select food and beverages for our weekly shopping most of us trust, and expect, that the contents of the packets of food packages on display will match the information on the labels. The source of the food is something we rarely question, but is everything we eat and drink really what we think it is?

Fighting Food Fraud

Food fraud and adulteration were first addressed in the USA by food law as far back as 1784. The FDA, in the 19th century, began protecting consumers from snake oil salesman and other charlatans that preyed on the susceptible public with their alchemy–spiked tonic and elixirs. To help counter this now, the FDA has several hundred agents deployed worldwide as part of its chemical investigations division to investigate food fraud.

One of the main reasons that food fraud does not get as much attention as it deserves is because the effects on the human body usually go unnoticed, or the connection between illness and fraudulent–food consumption is not clear. As a result, the scale of food fraud is unknown. Dressing up food ingredients is a common practice worldwide.

The Top Ten most adulterated foods in the United States in 2013 were:

- olive oil
- milk
- honey
- saffron
- orange juice
- coffee
- apple juice
- grape wine
- vanilla extract
- and maple syrup.

For consumers who cook with olive oil, the food safety threat is tremendous. The reason being olive oil is often diluted with peanut oil. If a consumer has a peanut allergy, it becomes a profoundly serious, even life–threatening situation. By the time food adulteration is uncovered, the health effects have already happened. If those effects are severe allergic reactions or organ failure, it is too late.

It is true that most food fraud cases do not typically lead to widespread outbreaks, but that does not negate the fact that food fraud is potentially dangerous and poses a very real public health concern. In the early 1980s, hundreds of people died from contaminated cooking oil in Spain. More recently, in China the industrial chemical "melamine" was found in powdered baby milk, leading to fatalities and thousands of infants falling ill.

Over the past decades, food supply chains have grown increasingly complex and many of today's food products repeatedly cross national boundaries, creating more opportunities for criminals to practice food fraud.

Coaching Consumers

Of course, any conversation on food safety and food fraud must include the consumer. The role that consumers play is a big issue for Consumers International, the world federation of consumer groups. While manufacturers have a responsibility to ensure food safety and uses traceability to guarantee the origin of food Ingredients, consumers bear much responsibility for awareness and safety.

A study released by the National Center of Biotechnology Information, whose mission is to contribute to the National Institute of Health's mission of 'uncovering new knowledge,' in 2013 touches on several factors that dictate food choices. According to the literature, very few Americans consume diets that meet the recommendations of the 2010 Dietary Guidelines for Americans. The complexity of the food and information environments makes it difficult for all consumers to improve their dietary patterns. This calls for nutrition education to give individuals the knowledge and skills necessary to navigate these environments in a way that results in healthful food choices.

Another driving factor in nutritional choices is level of education. A study released by University of Pennsylvania showed the higher the education levels of a U.S. household, the healthier the foods its members buy. Education levels, as opposed to income levels or access to supermarkets, determine food preferences. Based on the findings of this study, wealth, and education, not access, drives healthy food choices.

Crushing Food Fears

There is concerning data that reveals declining consumer trust in food and beverage companies. According to a 2020 study, fewer than one in four consumers in the U.S. trust labels on food packaging. What is more, younger Americans have more skepticism than older generations and hold higher ethical standards for brands.

Clean labels with recognizable ingredients rank highly, though many shoppers want to go a step further. Consumers do not want food companies to be "secret and opaque," according to a recent survey, meaning they want to know exactly what is in their food, not necessarily what is not. They also want to know how ingredients are sourced and how their health might be affected.   This concept incorporates a form of food traceability where the origin of the food is identified to consumers.

Chapter 13: The Nice List?

What does 'all natural' really mean? When people want to get healthier, they make a conscious decision to buy healthier foods at the grocery store, or at least what they think are healthier foods. But unfortunately, the reality is many people are getting duped by misleading package labeling.

As a consumer, you may be interested in buying the healthiest foods you can find, which means you will be gleaning nutrition and health information from food labels. Two sources of information include the nutrition facts label and the ingredients list located on the back or side of the packaging.

In addition to those required labels, you may find a host of health or nutrition claims made on the front of the packaging. One common claim is "natural," "all natural," or "made with natural Ingredients." What does it mean when food manufacturers' use these terms?

According to Merriam Webster Dictionary, the definition of "natural" that fits the food world best is "closely resembling an original: true to nature." So, all-natural foods should be those that are closest to their pure, natural state. However, it is hard to imagine any processed food as being close to its natural state, as most Ingredients have undergone some kind of alteration before being placed on store shelves.

The belief, of course, is that something that is "all natural" is going to be much better for you than something that contains artificial ingredients. While that may be true, seeing the word "natural" on a food product may not mean what you hope it means. Folic acid, for example, is an artificial form of B vitamin that is beneficial.

What the FDA Says About 'Natural'

The FDA decides what types of health and nutrition claims can be put on packaged foods. For example, the FDA has requirements for using the phrase "low fat" on a food label. Unfortunately, the FDA does not have an official definition for natural foods, so their official position on using the word "natural" is that the term is appropriate if the food does not contain added colors, artificial flavors, or synthetic substances.

Without any formal regulation, the consumer is left to trust the food manufacturers. A food product that is made with "all-natural" ingredients could still contain hormones, be genetically modified, or be filled with harmful substances many consumers worry about. Natural foods do not have to be organically produced, and it does not mean the farm animals were treated well. All-natural foods can also be high in calories, fats, sodium, or sugar.

In short, if you see the words "all natural" on a food package, you still need to do a little digging to truly know if the product is good for you and your family.

What a "natural" food label really means

As previously mentioned, the FDA states a product may be deemed natural if it does not contain any artificial or synthetic additives or ingredients. It further states that any product containing an ingredient that would not typically be found in that product cannot brandish the label. However, this does not encompass any sort of processing, like pasteurization, irradiation, or use of pesticides. As a result, a product subjected to such procedures can still be labeled as natural.

The USDA, on the other hand, has a legal definition for "natural", but it applies only to meat and poultry, containing no artificial ingredients or added colors, and is only minimally processed. Minimal processing means that the product was processed in a manner that does not fundamentally alter the product.

Most people are misled by food labels

Seasoned organic shoppers and health experts may be aware of these fuzzy guidelines, but average consumers are not. According to a recent Consumer Report survey that polled Americans on what they think natural on a food label means, more than 80% of people agreed that a "natural" label should mean that a product 'is not made with synthetic chemicals, artificial additives or colors, toxic pesticides, and genetically modified organisms.' We now know, based on previous information, that this is not the case.

The idea of buying "all-natural" foods may seem like a good idea, but since the FDA does not regulate the use of the word, you will need to examine the ingredients list and the nutrition facts labels to find the healthiest packaged foods. Meaning, the ownness of information is on the consumer.

Is Organic Better?

Amidst nutrition facts, ingredient lists, and dietary claims on food packages, "organic" might appear as one more piece of information to decipher when shopping for products. Understanding what the organic label means can help shoppers make informed purchasing choices.

According to USDA, Organic is a labeling term found on products that have been produced using cultural, biological, and mechanical practices that support the cycling of on-farm resources, promote ecological balance, and conserve biodiversity. The National Organic Program enforces the organic regulations, ensuring the integrity of the USDA Organic Seal.

To make an organic claim or use the USDA Organic Seal, the final product must follow strict production, handling and labeling standards and go through the organic certification process. The standards address a variety of factors such as soil quality, animal raising practices, as well as pest and weed control. Synthetic fertilizers, sewage sludge, irradiation, and genetic engineering may not be used.

Organic producers rely on natural substances and physical, mechanical, or biologically based farming methods to the fullest extent possible. Organic produce must be grown on soil that had no prohibited substances, most synthetic fertilizers, and pesticides, applied for three years prior to harvest. As for organic meat, the standards require that animals are raised in living conditions accommodating their natural behaviors, fed organic feed, and not administered antibiotics or hormones.

There are four distinct labeling categories for organic products – 100 percent organic, organic, "made with" organic ingredients, and specific organic ingredients.

In the "100 Percent Organic" category, products must be made up of 100 percent certified organic ingredients. The label must include the name of the certifying agent and may include the USDA Organic Seal and/or the 100 percent organic claim.

In the "Organic" category, the product and ingredients must be certified organic, except where specified on National List of Allowed and Prohibited Substances. Non-organic ingredients allowed per the National List may be used, but no more than five percent of the combined total ingredients may contain non-organic content. Additionally, the label must include the name of the certifying agent and may include the USDA Organic Seal and/or the organic claim.

For multi-ingredient products in the "made with" organic category, at least 70 percent of the product must be certified organic ingredients. The organic seal cannot be used on the product, and the final product cannot be represented as organic – only up to three ingredients or ingredient categories can be represented as organic. Any remaining ingredients are not required to be organically produced but must be produced without excluded methods- genetic engineering. All non-agricultural products must be allowed on the National List. For example, processed organic foods may contain some approved non-agricultural ingredients, like enzymes in yogurt, pectin in fruit jams, or baking soda in baked goods.

Multi-ingredient products with less than 70 percent certified organic content would fall under the "specific organic ingredients," and do not need to be certified. These products cannot display the USDA Organic Seal or use the word organic on the principal display panel. They can list certified organic ingredients in the ingredient list and the percentage of organic ingredients.

Becoming familiar with organic labeling allows consumers to make informed decisions about the products they purchase. Consumers can be assured that the integrity of USDA organic products are verified from farm to market.

Chapter 14: Clean Fifteen

Most of us understand that organic produce is the best choice, but some struggle with the impact of an all-organic diet on their monthly budget. That is where the EWG, or Environmental Working Group's, "Shopper's Guide to Pesticides in Produce," comes in.

There are certain fruits and vegetables that carry a higher load of pesticides, herbicides, and insecticides, while others have lower levels of toxic residues. The guide ranks 48 popular fruits and vegetables based on an analysis of 34,000 samples tested by the U.S. Department of Agriculture and the federal Food and Drug Administration. Note: The USDA does not test every food every year, so the EWG uses the most recent sampling period for each food.

The goal of this list is to help us eat healthier and reduce exposure by providing us a list of produce that is the most contaminated when grown under the presence of pesticides. For those who cannot or do not desire to make a 100% organic switch, these foods should always be substituted with organic choices to minimize ingestion of potentially dangerous chemicals. This list helps maximize healthy choices while minimizing the financial impact.

The List
1. Avocado
2. Sweet Corn
3. Pineapple
4. Onion
5. Papaya
6. Sweet Peas Frozen
7. Eggplant
8. Asparagus
9. Cauliflower
10. Cantaloupes
11. Broccoli
12. Mushrooms

13. Cabbage
14. Honeydew Melon
15. Kiwi

Chapter 15: Making healthier food choices

In the absence of strict rules and guidelines regarding food manufacturers 'claims' about their products, how can one make healthier choices? Furthermore, how can one be clear they're choices are, in fact, healthier? Doing a little research about various products before you head to the store can help you make more informed decisions when you get there. And knowing which labels to look for, and what they mean, can also help.

Here are some things to keep in mind:

- Look for food certifications, not just the color of the packaging. Green color does not equal clean or natural.
- Look for the '100% USDA Organic' seal.
- 'Free range' or 'grass-fed' labels. Do not just trust the label. Do some research around specific company practices before buying at the store.
- Consider purchasing from local farmers where claims can be vetted.

Ingredients that seem healthy but should be reconsidered:

- 'Whole grain' or 'multigrain.' Look for the '100% Whole Grain' stamp.
    - Multigrain: Though it sounds like a healthy choice, there is no guarantee that multigrain bread is made with 100 percent whole grains, nor that it is free of refined grains. It simply means that it contains more than one type of grain, such as wheat, oats, and quinoa. These grains may have been processed to remove their bran and germ, which strips them of nutritional value (including fiber and important nutrients). Because of this, it may not be as healthy as whole grain or whole wheat bread. Read the ingredient list and

look out for terms like "bleached" or "enriched," which means the bread is not made up entirely of whole grains.

- o Wheat bread: Wheat bread should *not* be confused with whole wheat bread. Wheat bread means the product is made using wheat flour, which is another term for refined white flour.
- o Partially hydrogenated oils: These oils contain trans fatty acids. These trans fats upset the balance between the good and bad cholesterol levels in your body, by both raising the bad and lowering the good. This ratio has been linked to a myriad of lifestyle diseases, including heart disease, stroke, and type 2 diabetes.

Eating for health: Ditch The cravings

Beyond the physiological reasons for food cravings, they often have something to do with emotion and desire. Eating junk food may be linked to an increase in depression. Cravings can have many harmful effects on you, like:

1. Weight gain. Eating excessive amounts of sugar, processed foods, fatty foods, drinking alcohol, and consuming salt can add extra pounds to even the healthiest person.
2. Health issues. Salty and fatty foods can both lead to high blood pressure and high cholesterol. Sugary foods like diet soft drinks can lead to heart attacks, dangerous blood clots and other cardiovascular problems.
3. Alcohol cravings. Craving alcohol can lead to physical problems like liver disease, gout, cancer, pancreatitis, and the immune system.
4. Dental problems. Sugary, processed foods as well as alcohol can all lead to dental problems ranging from tooth decay to gum disease.
5. Psychological issues. Trying to control your craving for certain foods and not being able to stop can lead to thoughts

of low self-esteem, believing something is wrong with you and other thought issues.

The Food Network offers these tips to help overcome food cravings.

Avoid your triggers
It is understood that you crave what you eat. If you change what you eat to what you want to crave, you will eradicate your "bad" food cravings for "good" ones. Gradually cutting out and avoiding what you are craving helps you to begin to want them less.

Do away with temptation
Go through your kitchen pantry and get rid of all the foods that you crave. If you bought a box of cookies on your last shopping trip, throw them out, or give them away.

Munch on nuts
Eat an ounce of nuts with two glasses of water to help you overcome your craving. The crunch will satisfy your need to chew, and the water will make you feel full.

Let go of stress
Stress is a huge reason for cravings. Learning how to reduce and deal with the daily stress in your life can help you overcome food cravings. Look for different techniques like deep breathing or exercising that can help.

Chapter 16: Grocery Shopping 101

No matter how discerning your palate, chances are you have been fooled a time or two when shopping for food at the supermarket. And unlike the counterfeit wallet or handbag bought on the streets of New York City, this bit of fakery is under the radar. It could have been those pricey heirloom tomatoes or that bottle of imported extra virgin olive oil. Someone, somewhere along the supply chain pulled a switcheroo. The heirlooms were really garden variety tomatoes. The extra virgin olive oil was cut with hazelnut oil or a blend of lesser quality olive oils rather than a first pressing of Mediterranean olives. You want to think you would be able to tell the difference. But "the perpetrators are not designing these changes to be detected," says Karen Everstine, a research associate at the University of Minnesota's Food Protection and Defense Institute and the group's resident food fraud expert. "And presumably, most of the time, they aren't."

The following are some tips to aid you in your journey to begin your transition:

Never Go Hungry

If you are going into a physical store then this should really be rule #1! If you arrive at the grocery store with a hungry tummy, you may be more tempted to give in to processed snacks and food cravings. It may lead us to want instantaneous satisfaction, making us more likely to shop for processed packaged foods that can be opened and eaten right away or lead us to either the prepared food section or worse, the middle isles. Do your will power a favor and make your trip to the grocery store after having a healthy bite to eat.

Eating healthy means eating more raw fruits and vegetables. This, in turn, means more frequent grocery shopping to assist in ensuring food bought today stays fresh longer. Pay attention to dates.

Always Check Dates - and Understand the Lingo

The worst part about buying fresh produce is getting home and realizing it expires tomorrow! Before you stock your shopping cart with chicken, beef, turkey, yogurt, milk, always check the expiration date. The following information will aid you in understanding package labeling where freshness is concerned.

- Best By: This is a recommendation and has nothing to do with safety. It is there to tell customers when a product should be eaten for ideal quality, preserving maximizing taste and texture.
- Sell By: This date is aimed at retailers. It shows what date an item should be sold by or when it should be removed from the shelf. It is not a safety indicator and often you will see items in the clearance section, being sold at a reduced cost because of being past this date.
- Use By: This is a recommendation and has nothing to do with safety, except when used on infant formula according to USDA. It is there to tell customers when a product should be eaten for ideal quality, preserving maximizing taste and texture.
- Freeze By: Another label that, according to the USDA, has nothing to do with safety. Rather, it indicates when a product should be frozen to maintain peak quality.

Grab Food From the Back of the Shelf
When stockers load groceries onto the shelves, they usually place the newest items in the back. This helps to ensure a first-in/first-out turnover on food, ensuring those items with shortest shelf life sell first. Thus, if you're looking for the freshest foods that will last the longest amount of time in your fridge, your best bet is to reach to the back.

Go for Quality!
If you're really trying to bump up your healthy eating game, it is not only important to think about what you eat, but also where your

food comes from. While organic produce, grass-fed meats, and wild-caught fish may cost more, they do have their benefits.

Chill Out: Do not Be Afraid of Frozen Veggies
Frozen foods often get a bad rap, but frozen fruits and veggies are usually picked at their peak ripeness. As a result, they are generally packed with the most nutrients. Depending on what you are craving and what season it is, frozen produce may be fresher than what you find in the produce sections. Additionally, as a bonus if you see frozen fruits or vegetables on sale, feel free to load up. While they may end up freezer burnt if left for a long enough period, they will not spoil. Not to mention, they last so much longer than their fresh counterparts.

What is freezer burn? Freezer burn is moisture loss. It is not a pathogen and has nothing to do with food safety, just food quality. But when it happens to otherwise perfectly good food, it's a bummer because freezer burnt food is just not tasty. An effective way to help prevent, besides consuming in a timely manner, is to make sure all the air is removed from opened packaging before placing into the freezer and ensure it is sealed tight.

The Middle Aisles
Most of us have heard the advice to shop around the perimeter of the grocery store and avoid the middle aisles to make healthier choices when shopping. Unfortunately, that's not exactly the case these days. Grocery stores seem to have caught on and have done some rearranging. The adage of "shop the perimeter" is simply no longer true.

Some traditional departments around the edges of the grocery store have never been healthy, the bakery for example. Whilst the perimeter is where you usually find fresh fruit, vegetables, dairy, and fresh meats, skipping the middle aisles can mean missing out on a range of healthy food products. These foods can aid in simplifying healthy eating and making it more convenient, from canned sardines to dried soup lentils. Keep in mind that temptation does lurk in the middle aisles, so it is best to have a list and to stick to it.

Some guiding principles
Keep in mind that the primary goal here is to choose food as close to its natural form as possible. Look for whole, fresh food and minimize or eliminate processed foods. The more highly processed the food is, the worse it is for our health. This will require some time, patience and sleuthing to find the best choices for you and your family.

Produce
A study by Reuse This Bag showed that produce from a traditional grocery store contains about 746 times more bacteria than a car's steering wheel. Grocery stores themselves are rife with bacteria, from the carts to the refrigerator doors. Reusable produce bags, while it is a commendable thing to do, are also potentially introducing even more bacteria to your produce, since carts from traditional grocery stores have nearly 361 times more bacteria than a bathroom doorknob. Another place that is bad for naked produce is the checkout lane's conveyor belt. It is advised by grocery insiders to never place loose produce on the belt, especially on busy days. Those belts get dirty and can be contaminated with residue and bacteria from meat, amongst other things. Studies by the International Association of Food Protection show that yeast, mold, staph, and coliforms are living and growing on these belts. Unfortunately, these belts are porous, so you can scrub them day and night, but you can never get them fully clean.

Thoroughly wash fruits and vegetables before cooking or eating them. Produce that the manufacturer has prewashed does not require further rinsing, however, there are two main risks of eating unwashed fruits and vegetables: bacterial contamination and pesticides.

Another case for why it is always a good reason to religiously wash your berries, one insider leaked, "If we spilled the berries on the floor in the back room, we just packed them all back in the package and put them back on the shelf without cleaning them." Another worker echoed this sentiment for all fruit, saying, "Clean your fruits before you eat them, more often than not they've been on the very dirty floor."

On another note, the reason grocery store produce like apples and cucumbers are super shiny is not because of some superior farming practice. It is because they are coated in wax. Some produce does have a natural wax, but even then, it still might get coated in additional food-grade wax to help it stay fresh, retain moisture, and inhibit mold growth. According to the FDA, it is perfectly safe to eat, though the human body cannot digest it. Waxes simply pass through our digestive systems untouched. And since the wax is made to be water-repellant, you cannot just rinse it off, meaning unless you peel the fruit where most of the nutrients are, it is getting eaten.

Meat
Most of the meat purchased at supermarkets comes from livestock that has been raised on what are called Concentrated Animal Feeding Operations, also known as "factory farms."

There are about 257,000 of these factory farms in the United States, and the EPA defines them as "a production process that concentrates large numbers of animals in relatively small and confined places, and that substitutes structures and equipment (for feeding, temperature controls, and manure management) for land and labor."

Animals kept in these conditions will not typically be healthy, so antibiotics, hormones, de-worming medication, growth-promoting drugs, and other medicines that help them reach their slaughter weight quickly and without getting too sick become the norm.

According to a recent USDA Inspector General Report, beef sold to the public was found to be contaminated with 211 different drug residues.

While many countries have protections against salmonella in place at chicken farms and hatcheries, there are no such protections in the U.S., where testing is only carried out on a limited basis at the slaughterhouse. Here, it's simply accepted that chicken will have potentially fatal bacteria on it. According to federal data, about 25 percent of raw chicken pieces contain salmonella, as a result, nearly 200,000 Americans are sickened with salmonella from poultry annually. In 2016, the USDA finalized new food safety measures to reduce salmonella.

Dairy/Milk
Milk is a staple item that ends up in almost everyone's shopping cart. Even if you are vegan, chances are you are at least buying cartons of almond or coconut milk. Paying attention, one might notice that this area is nearly always in the furthest back corner of the store, typically as far away from the front doors as possible.

Why is that?? Well, it is not an accident. For decades, savvy grocery store owners, managers, and companies have known that all shoppers will seek this department out. If they placed this are near the front doors, some shoppers would undoubtedly grab their milk and go. But, if shoppers must virtually walk through the entire store, they are much more likely to pick up a few extra things along the way.

Ugly truth about milk
A 2012 report published in the *Archives of Pediatric and Adolescent Medicine* authored by Kendrin Sonneville from Harvard University tracked fracture rates in 6,712 adolescents. The results showed that active children who consumed the largest quantities of milk had more bone fractures than those who consumed less. Thus, contrary to the myth, *milk does not actually build strong bones.*

Studies of young women published in the journals *Bone* and *Pediatrics* show that bone density was reinforced by physical activity, but that increased calcium intake made no difference. Similarly, a Harvard study of 20,885 men published in 2001 showed that men having 2_1/2 servings of dairy products daily had a 34% increased risk of prostate cancer, compared with men consuming little or no dairy products. A separate Harvard study, including 47,871 men, yielded similar results. Men having two or more milk servings each day had a 60% increased risk of prostate cancer.

The scientific issue of most concern to public health officials is the load of fat in dairy products. The 2010 Dietary Guidelines for Americans described the main source of fat, that leads to heart disease and other health problems in the American diet, to be saturated fat or the "bad" fat. Dairy products turned out to be the biggest source of these fats. Typical cheeses are about 70% fat, much of which is saturated fat. Skimming the fat from milk leaves a drink loaded with sugar. Lactose sugar contributes more than 55% of skim milk's calories, giving it a calorie load like soda.

Surprisingly cow's milk consumption by infants and toddlers is linked to type 1 diabetes and to anemia. As children reach their teen years, many experience cramps and diarrhea due to lactose intolerance.

Yogurt
While yogurt has some healthy benefits, the correct choice here can be tricky section. Watch for added sugar and fat. Greek yogurt is higher in protein and almost always a better choice. It is best to choose plain versions and add your own fresh or frozen fruit.

Cheese
Cheese is a great source of protein and calcium but is often high in saturated fat and salt. If you venture to this section, seek out lower fat, "real" cheese options and avoid processed cheese product/food.

Even though lower fat cheese is a better option than regular, it is still a relatively high-fat food and should be consumed sparingly. Recent studies have shown that consuming too much cheese can lead to high cholesterol, high blood pressure, heart disease, diabetes, and stroke. Cheese is not the miracle food we have all been brought up to believe. In fact, many people are lactose intolerant and lack the digestive enzymes to break down cheese and other dairy products.

Cereal
Breakfast cereals are highly processed, often packed with added sugar and refined carbs. Their packages regularly have misleading health claims. Breakfast cereals are marketed as healthy with boxes featuring health claims like "low-fat" and "whole-grain." Yet, the first listed ingredients are often refined grains and sugar.

Most breakfast cereals are loaded with sugar and refined grains, and high sugar consumption is harmful and may increase your risk of several diseases. Breakfast cereal is made from processed grains and often fortified with vitamins and minerals. Despite this, breakfast cereals are marketed under the guise of being healthy.

The process of making cereal is typically the following steps:
1. **Processing:** The grains are usually processed into fine flour and cooked.
2. **Mixing:** The flour is then mixed with ingredients like sugar, cocoa, and water.
3. **Extrusion:** Many breakfast cereals are produced via extrusion. Extrusion is a high-temperature process that uses a machine to shape the cereal.
4. **Drying:** Next, the cereal is dried.
5. **Shaping:** Finally, the cereal is shaped into forms, such as balls, stars, loops or rectangles.

Breakfast cereals may also be puffed, flaked, shredded, or coated in chocolate or frosting before it is dried. Loaded with sugar and refined carbs, most cereals list sugar as the second or third ingredient. Thus, starting the day with a high-sugar breakfast cereal will spike your blood sugar and insulin levels. Preparing a healthy breakfast from whole foods is not only simple but starts your day with plenty of nutrition.

Bread
The highly processed flour and additives in white, packaged bread can make it unhealthful. Consuming too much white bread can contribute to obesity, heart disease, and diabetes. Foods made from highly processed grains cause blood sugar to spike soon after eating. Frequent blood sugar spikes can eventually contribute to the development of type 2 diabetes. A high intake of simple carbohydrates, such as premade white bread, can lead to weight gain and a higher risk for diabetes, heart disease, and other lifestyle-related chronic conditions.

Processed carbs also lack fiber. As a result, a person will not feel full after eating them. They will crave more food again soon after, especially when the blood sugar drops. When manufacturers process foods, it often results in the loss of nutrients. The producers often add vitamins and minerals to white bread to replace these missing nutrients. However, they cannot replace the fiber, which is essential for digestive and cardiovascular health.

Buying bread with the word "whole" as the first ingredient still does not guarantee a healthful product though it improves the likelihood. Many types of bread contain added sugars or sugar substitutes. Even whole-grain bread can contain 20 or more ingredients, including preservatives and added salt and sugars. Not all of these contribute to good health. Preservatives may help bread stay fresh for longer, however fresh bread that contains fewer preservatives can be stored in the refrigerator or freezer to maintain freshness.

Bread made with sprouted grains is a good option. When a grain is sprouted, its nutrients become easier to digest and more available to the body for use. It can be a better source of protein, fiber, vitamin C, folate, and other nutrients. The whole grains in whole wheat bread have many benefits. They can boost overall health and help reduce the risk of obesity and various other complications and diseases.

The Whole Grains Council defines whole foods as one that contains all the essential parts and naturally occurring nutrients of the entire grain seed in their original proportions. If the grain has been processed, i.e., cracked, crushed, rolled, extruded, or cooked, the food product should deliver the same rich balance of nutrients that are found in the original grain seed.

Pasta
Most people prefer refined pasta, meaning that the wheat kernel has been stripped of the germ and bran along with many of the nutrients it contains.
Refined pasta is higher in calories and lower in fiber. This may result in decreased feelings of fullness after you eat it, compared to eating high-fiber, whole-grain pasta.

According to a federal study of more than 117,000 people, a link between a high carb intake and an increased risk of heart disease was revealed, especially when the intake was from refined grains. Another study of a little more than 2,000 people found that higher refined grain consumption was associated with increased waist circumference, blood pressure, blood sugar, bad LDL cholesterol, blood triglycerides and insulin resistance. It is important to note, however, that the glycemic index of pasta is in the low to medium range, which is lower than that of many other processed foods. Thus, it is the lesser of many evils.

Eating whole grains has been associated with a lower risk of heart disease, colorectal cancer, diabetes, and obesity. Whole grains are made from the entire wheat kernel. As a result, they are higher in fiber, vitamins, and minerals than refined grains, which contain only the endosperm of the wheat kernel. Keep in mind that whole-grain pasta is made from whole-wheat flour that has been pulverized. This process diminishes the beneficial effects of the whole grains found in pasta since grains with smaller particles are digested more rapidly, leading to greater increases in blood sugar. Therefore, the benefits of pasta made from whole grains are not comparable to the benefits of intact whole grains, such as oats, brown rice, or quinoa.

Still, while there is little difference in the effects of refined and whole-grain pastas on health, pasta that is made from whole grains may be a better choice if you are looking to lose weight. It is lower in calories and higher in satiety boosting, fiber than refined pasta. Satiety boosting nutrients are digested slowly in our bodies, providing longer-lasting feelings of fullness. High satiety foods prevent that spike in blood sugar and the resulting crash, which leads to feelings of hunger and cravings. Whole-grain pasta contains a higher amount of most micronutrients, aside from B vitamins, which are added back into enriched pasta during processing.

Seafood
While eating fish has nutritional benefits, it also has potential risks. Fish can take in harmful chemicals from the water and the food they eat. Substances like mercury and PCBs can build up in their bodies over time. High levels of mercury and PCBs can harm the brain and nervous system.

In one study, exposure to mercury stood out as the main risk factor for autoimmunity. Autoimmune disease, which can include such conditions as inflammatory bowel disease, lupus, Sjogren's syndrome, rheumatoid arthritis, and multiple sclerosis, is among the ten leading causes of death among women, the study noted. Greater exposure to mercury was associated with a higher rate of autoantibodies, a precursor to autoimmune disease.

The American Heart Association recommends people eat 2 servings of fatty fish each week. Fish such as swordfish, king mackerel and tilefish contain the highest levels of mercury. Healthier options include fresh (not canned) tuna, herring, mackerel, salmon, sardines, and trout.

Around the perimeter
This is where you will find the freshest foods, including produce, meat, and dairy. Fresh foods are generally healthier than the processed foods you will find in the center aisles. With the appropriate intake of fruits and vegetables, one can better control the fat and sodium intake in your diet. Maintaining a healthy diet means watching what is added to foods, as well. Many foods in the center aisles contain preservatives. If foods do not have any added preservatives, then they need to be refrigerated to keep fresh. The goal is to have three quarters of the cart filled with items around the perimeter, or the outside part of the store. If followed, there is less available space in the cart to add items from the middle aisles, where a great deal of the higher calorie and preservative filled items tend to lurk.

Success. Now that a foundation has been laid for label reading, making better choices, and improving on your health and emotional wealth, what is the best way to achieve success? There is a short answer and that is meal prep. There are few healthy options if you are busy and on the go, so meal prep is key. Having an idea of the foods that you will be cooking and the meals that you intend on having for the week will aid in success on this journey towards healthier eating. This is the first step in the journey. Once the menu has been established, bring the ingredients list with you to the store. It is easy to over shop, or buy unhealthy items in the grocery store if we do not have a clear direction. With focus, one can successfully load up the grocery cart, utilizing the tools learned in this read, and put thought to action.

It is worth the effort. Navigating the grocery store can feel overwhelming, especially at the beginning of a healthy lifestyle change, but give it some time. Be patient with yourself and make it a family affair. Slow changes are best and more likely to stick. Once you have nailed down the right foods for your family, it will get easier.

Recap

To some, grocery shopping may be an exciting weekly outing to pick up our favorite fruits, vegetables, and ingredients for our weekly meal prep. For others, it may be an overwhelming chore. grocery stores, bright, colorful, and full of options, can actually be more deceiving than we think. Truth be told, branding and product placement play huge factors in our grocery shopping experience. Some stores are even paid extra to house certain products at a proper eye and hand distance away, in the hopes that customers are more likely to drop the items into their carts.

Read the labels. Do not be persuaded by fancy packaging while grocery shopping. It is especially important to read the labels on the food that you're purchasing. A general rule of thumb: If you can not pronounce the ingredient name (or the Ingredients list is rather long), you probably should not be eating it too much. Sneaky preservatives and refined sugars can be hidden in our everyday foods. Unless we flip over our purchases and read the ingredients labels, we will never know.

Bring the clean fifteen and dirty dozen list with you. Not all fruits and vegetables are created equal when it comes to the number of harmful pesticides farmers spray on their crops.

Keep it colorful. When you look down at your grocery cart what do you see? Is it a basket full of boxes and packaged foods, or colorful fruits and veggies? At a minimum, there should be at least five different colors. Due to the number of nutrients varying amongst colored fruits and veggies, it is a safe bet to assume that the different colors attribute to varieties of vitamins and minerals, helping to prevent certain types of illness, including cancer and heart disease.

Now that we have established the importance food has in our life, it is time to discuss digestion. Let us take a look inside the toilet and have a chat.

Chapter 17: The Scoop on Poop

Since the day you were born, you had to eat, breathe and excrete waste in order to survive. When we eat and digest food, our bodies take in nutrition. It keeps what it needs through the absorption of nutrients and expels the rest. This is what keeps the body functioning properly and efficiently.

As off-putting as it may be to talk poop, paying attention to your excrement can tune you in to your overall health. From the color, shape, size, and smell of your poop, you can tell you a lot about what is going on inside your body, your cellular functions. Therefore, it is extremely important to pay attention.

Our bowel movements are typically made up of organic matter, good bacteria and bile, a chemical from the liver that helps digest fat, that our body no longer needs and thus, must be removed. When it comes to poop there is no universal standard for what is considered normal.

What is "normal?"

Everyone's normal is different. According to the experts, the frequency, texture, and smell of each person's bowel movement is as unique as the individual. The idea that pooping daily is a requirement for good health is a myth. For some, three a day is normal, for others three to four times a week is "normal." This is barring there are no complaints regarding digestion issues. Diet plays a very large role in not only frequency, but also texture, size, shape, and smell. Outside of what you eat, exercise, sleep deprivation, water intake, hormonal fluctuations, menopause, and medications can all influence your bowel movements.

According to WebMD, your digestive system is remarkably efficient. In the space of a few hours, it extracts nutrients from the foods you eat and drink, processes them into the bloodstream, and prepares leftover material for disposal. That material passes through about twenty feet of intestine before being stored temporarily in the colon, where water is removed. The residue is excreted through the bowels, normally within a day or two.

Depending on your diet, age, and daily activity, regularity can mean anything from three bowel movements a day to three each week. As fecal material sits in the colon, the harder the stool becomes and the more difficult it is to pass. A normal stool should not be either unusually hard or soft, and you should not have to strain unreasonably to pass it.

Fecal matter is 75 percent water and 25 percent solid matter, consisting of dead bacteria, indigestible food, and inorganic substances. It usually takes about three days for food to pass through your system, resulting in a bowel movement. But when food passes through your system too quickly or too slowly, it can affect the size, color, and texture of your stool.

Medical professionals use something called the Bristol Chart, see chart on next page, to classify bowel movements. The chart identifies seven categorizes, or types. Types 1 and 2 indicate constipation, 3 and 4 are the most ideal poops, and 5, 6, and 7 suggest diarrhea. Generally, most of us excrete type 3 or 4 feces. They are soft, formed, and easy to pass without the need to strain.

Bristol Stool

Type 1		Seperate hard lumps (Very constipated)
Type 2		Lumpy and sausage like (Slightly constipated)
Type 3		A sausage shape with cracks in the surface (Normal)
Type 4		Like a smooth, soft sausage or snake (Normal)
Type 5		Soft blobs with clear-cut edges (Lacking fibre)
Type 6		Mushy consistency with ragged edges (Inflammation)
Type 7		Liquid consistency with no solid pieces (Inflammation and diarrhea)

Eating a diet that is rich in fiber helps bulk up the stool, since fiber acts like a sponge to help retain some water. The American Academy of Family Physicians encourages nine servings per day of high fiber foods like fruits, vegetables, and legumes to help keep things running smoothly. Taking supplemental bulking agents like psyllium can also help to create large, soft stools that pass through the intestines smoothly and at a normal pace.

Dehydration is one of the most common causes of chronic constipation. This is because the intestines pull water into the bowels to make the stool softer and easier to pass. If you do not have enough water in your body already, the large intestine soaks up water from your food waste. This makes you have hard stools that are difficult to pass.

Food sensitivities, overgrowth of bacteria/yeast in the small intestine, and excessive intake of red meat or alcohol are also contributors to constipation. In addition to what one eats, traveling, various medications, lack of exercise, diseases like irritable bowel syndrome or Chrons, and pregnancy are all contributors to chronic constipation.

On the opposite end of the spectrum, many people have diarrhea on a regular basis, and far more often than they realize. If experiencing loose, mushy, or watery stools at least 75 percent of the time, you have chronic diarrhea. The consistency may be soft separate blobs, fluffy pieces with ragged edges, or be completely watery with no solid pieces at all. As with constipation, fiber plays an important role when you are suffering from diarrhea for many of the same reasons previously mentioned.

Other potential causes for chronic diarrhea include an overgrowth of bacteria and yeast in the large intestine, food sensitivities, excess intake of high fat or greasy foods, the inability to sufficiently digest and absorb nutrients, and chronic stress or anxiety due to the strong gut-brain connection.

Pay attention to your poop. The idea of studying one's own bowel movements probably is not something we would like to think about. But the size, shape, and color of your poop is a great indication of what is happening in the rest of your body. There are many reasons why a bowel movement has the size, shape and surface it does. Changes can be because of dietary challenges or infection or other serious conditions. The more you know about how to read these signs, the healthier you will be.

 It is important for bowels to work well since they absorb nutrients, but they also keep out any foods, chemicals, and germs that could hurt your body. Here are five important signs to look for in your stool.

Color

It can be a variety colors, depending on the foods being consumed. Some shades of brown are considered normal. Other colors, like black or yellow, are not.

Black or dark green stool can be the side effect of iron supplements, medicines such as Pepto-Bismol, or eating black licorice or blueberries. The dark stool could mean there is bleeding in the small intestine. If you see bright red, it could mean you're bleeding from the lower part of the large intestine or rectum. Under such circumstances, it is highly recommended to seek medical advice.

According to online publication Step to Health, when stool is white or pale in color, it is an indication of a problem with one's biliary system, which consists of the pancreas, liver, and gallbladder. The brown color of your stool comes from the bile salts secreted by the liver. If stool is white, a liver infection may be the culprit If that is the case, this will slow the production of bile. It may also be an indication of a bile duct obstruction.

Shape

A change in stool shape can also be a cause for concern. Narrow and pencil-thin stools are thought by some to be a symptom of colon cancer. It is thought that the narrow shape might be a sign of the lower part of the colon being blocked.

Soft stool can also be a sign of a problem. If it sticks to the side of the toilet bowl, or is difficult to flush, it may indicate the presence of too much oil. A good way to remember this is to remember oil floats in water. If the stool looks like fat droplets, it can mean the body is not absorbing the fats properly. Diseases such as chronic pancreatitis stop the body from properly absorbing fat. Generally, stool that sinks or floats does not mean there is a problem, it is because of how much gas is in the stool.

Smell

Bowel movements generally have a strong odor, but particularly strange or foul bowel movements may be a sign of something out of the ordinary happening in your body.

Stool is made up of undigested food, bacteria, mucus, and dead cells. It may smell worse than usual because of certain bacteria or parasites.

Blood in your stool can come with a strange odor and poop with too much fat can smell worse than a normal bowel movement. Reasons for a foul smell could also include certain medications, having food stuck in the colon for too long, or an infection.

Constipation

Dry, hard stool, which is difficult to eliminate, and having bowel movements fewer than three times a week are both signs of constipation. More than 4 million Americans have frequent constipation and most people will have it at least once.

If it is ignored, constipation could lead to complications such as hemorrhoids or rectal bleeding. The best way to relieve symptoms is to follow a well-balanced, high-fiber diet, drink plenty of water, exercise regularly, and go to the bathroom when you feel the urge. Holding in a bowel movement can lead to added discomfort.

Diarrhea

Diarrhea happens when loose, watery stools pass through your bowels too quickly. Generally, it lasts one or two days and goes away on its own. It is a normal way for the body to get rid of toxic substances, like bacteria or viral infections, but if not careful, can lead to dehydration.

The color, regularity, and consistency of your bowel movements are not the only characteristics that can tip you off to what is going on inside your body. There is also a host of information available at the microscopic level. The bacteria inside your stool, which can be analyzed through laboratory tests provide a snapshot of the microbes living in your intestines. The range of bacteria in the gut may have implications for a range of health conditions.

Chapter 18: Eating for digestion

You do not have to overhaul your entire diet to get a big health boost. Here are five simple changes you can put into action today for high-impact results.

Load Up on Fruits and Veggies
You know fruits and vegetables are good for you, but did you know they should fill half your plate at every meal?

Daily goal: 2 cups of fruit and 2.5 cups of veggies.

Sound like a lot? Try topping your morning eggs with salsa. Yes, it counts! Chose to lunch on vegetable soup or a sandwich topped with sprouts, snack on a strawberry-banana smoothie, without the added sugar. Add chopped-up veggies to your ground turkey meat loaf or homemade pasta sauce.

Choose Better Fats
It is essential to eat some fats, though it is also harmful to eat too much. The fats you eat give your body energy that it needs to work properly. During exercise, your body uses calories from carbohydrates you have eaten. But after 20 minutes, exercise depends partially on calories from fat to keep you going.

According to the Cleveland Clinic, the dietary reference intake (DRI) for fat in adults is 20% to 35% of total calories from fat. That is about 44 grams to 77 grams of fat per day if you eat 2,000 calories a day. It is recommended to eat more of some types of fats because they provide health benefits. It is recommended to eat less of other types of fat due to the negative impact on health.

- Monounsaturated fat: 15% to 20%
- Polyunsaturated fat: 5% to 10%
- Saturated fat: less than 10%
- Trans fat: 0%
- Cholesterol: less than 300 mg per day

Saturated fats are generally solid or waxy at room temperature and come mostly from animal products, except for tropical oils. Taking in too much saturated fat is linked with raising levels of "bad" LDL cholesterol in the blood and increasing internal inflammation. Healthy adults should limit their saturated fat intake to no more than 10% of total calories. For a person eating a 2000 calorie diet, this would be 22 grams of saturated fat or less per day.

According to an online article published by Medical News Today, healthful high-fat foods are not something to shy away from. The body needs a certain amount of fat from food intake to aid hormone function, memory, and the absorption of specific nutrients.

The most healthful fats are monounsaturated and polyunsaturated fats, which include omega-3 and omega-6 fatty acids. Saturated and trans fats can raise your bad cholesterol level and your risk of heart disease. By cutting back on animal-based foods like butter, bacon, and untrimmed meats, as well as pantry staples like cookies and crackers, you can keep these at bay.

Drink Water
The notion of eight ounces of water is a longly held myth. At some point, many of us have been told that proper hydration requires us to consume copious amounts of water. The research has refuted the eight-glasses-a-day fable riding a wave of weak scientific literature. In fact, many of the groups behind the public push for over-hydration have been exposed as having a monetary interest in the fluid industry. Essentially, there is no solid evidence suggesting that this is, in fact, the right amount, but it is probably a good recommendation for a minimum amount. Depending on your lifestyle, body type, diet, age, and more, this will vary.

You might need more water than someone else. How much water you need also depends on:

- **Where you live.** You will need more water in hot, humid, or dry areas. You will also need more water if you live in the mountains or at a high altitude.
- **Your diet.** If you drink a lot of coffee and other caffeinated beverages you might lose more water through extra urination. You will likely also need to drink more water if your diet is high in salty, spicy, or sugary foods or if you do not consume a significant number of hydrating foods that are high in water like fresh or cooked fruits and vegetables.
- **The temperature or season.** You may need more water in warmer months than cooler ones due to perspiration.
- **Your environment.** If you spend more time outdoors in the sun or hot temperatures or in a heated room, you might feel thirstier faster.
- **How active you are.** If you are active during the day or walk or stand a lot, you will need more water than someone who's sitting at a desk. If you exercise or do any intense activity, you will need to drink more to cover water loss.
- **Your health.** If you have an infection or a fever, or if you lose fluids through vomiting or diarrhea, you will need to drink more water. If you have a health condition like diabetes you will also need more water. Some medications, like diuretics, will increase your need for adequate water intake.
- **Pregnant or breastfeeding.** If you are pregnant or nursing your baby, you will need to drink extra water to stay hydrated.

Drinking 0.5 ounces of water per pound of your body weight each day is more accurate thumb rule, especially if you are overweight. This includes fluids from water, beverages like teas and juice, and from food, as you get an average of 20 percent of your water from the foods you eat according to the Academy of Nutrition of Dietetics.

Roughly 60% of your body weight is made of water. You need it for every single body function. It flushes toxins from your organs, carries nutrients to your cells, cushions your joints, and helps you digest the food you eat. Urine color as your guide is an indication of proper hydration. The body constantly loses water throughout the day, mostly through urine and sweat but also from regular body functions like breathing. To prevent dehydration, you need to get plenty of water from drink and food every day.

Drinking enough water is required for your body to function in general. Several health problems may also respond well to increased water intake:

- **Constipation.** Increasing water intake can help with constipation, a quite common problem.
- **Urinary tract infections.** Recent studies have shown that increasing water consumption may help prevent recurring urinary tract and bladder infection.
- **Kidney stones.** An older study concluded that high fluid intake decreased the risk of kidney stones, though more research is needed.

- **Skin hydration.** Studies show that more water leads to better skin hydration, though more research is needed on improved clarity and effects on acne.

Eat Fiber

Fiber is either soluble, which dissolves in water, or insoluble, which does not dissolve.

Soluble fiber. This type of fiber dissolves in water to form a gel-like material. It can help lower blood cholesterol and glucose levels. Soluble fiber is found in oats, peas, beans, apples, citrus fruits, carrots, barley, and psyllium.

Insoluble fiber. This type of fiber promotes the movement of material through your digestive system and increases stool bulk, so it can be of benefit to those who struggle with constipation or irregular stools. Whole-wheat flour, wheat bran, nuts, beans, and vegetables, such as cauliflower, green beans, and potatoes, are good sources of insoluble fiber.

The amount of soluble and insoluble fiber varies in different plant foods. To receive the greatest health benefit, eat a wide variety of high-fiber foods. A high-fiber diet:

- Normalizes bowel movements.
- Helps maintain bowel health.
- Lowers cholesterol levels.
- Helps control blood sugar levels.
- Aids in achieving healthy weight.
- Helps you live longer.

Good fiber choices include:

- Whole-grain products
- Fruits
- Vegetables
- Beans, peas, and other legumes
- Nuts and seeds.

Refined or processed foods are lower in fiber. Examples are canned fruits and vegetables, pulp-free juices, white breads and pastas, and non-whole-grain cereals. Enriched foods have some of the B vitamins and iron added back after processing, but not the fiber that is lost in the grain-refining process, which removes the outer coat (bran) from the grain and lowers its fiber content.

Whole foods rather than fiber supplements are generally better. Fiber supplements, such as Metamucil, Citrucel and FiberCon, do not provide the variety of fibers, vitamins, minerals, and other beneficial nutrients that foods do.

Release the Toxins

We have become exposed to an increasing number of chemicals in our food supply, the air we breathe, and through many common items we use daily, including cosmetics and household cleaner. The WHO monitors the food and water supply for toxins and has found that a large percentage of food consumed by Americans is deemed unsafe. The highest concentration of toxins is derived from glycophosate. This is the chemical found in the pesticide Roundup. Roundup is commonly used to spray our agriculture, highways, parks, and playgrounds to kill weed.

Glycophosate is an antibiotic which kills a person's healthy microbiome. It binds to critical minerals, antioxidants, and vitamins and prevents them from being bioavailable. Some toxins can be absorbed through your skin. Personal care products, like shampoos, make-up, perfumes, and lotions often contain parabens, formaldehyde, and phenoxyethanol. As these products are absorbed, those toxins come into the body too. Some toxins come in through your supplements, toothpaste, and medications since many of them contain gelatin. Gelatin is often contaminated with misfolded proteins, or prions, that can trigger normal proteins in the brain to fold abnormally. These prions characterize several fatal and transmissible neurodegenerative diseases in humans and many other animals.

A body that is toxic has a two-fold problem. For starters, this vessel is holding on to fat cells. As a result, losing weight will be difficult at best. The second issue for anyone struggling with weight loss is that toxins also damage mitochondria, the energy powerhouses of the body. This leads to low energy and a sluggish metabolism, adding to the weight loss struggles. Even worse, toxins can also accumulate directly in the fatty lining of any cell in the body. This includes muscles, brain, nerves, skin, gut and more. This accumulation can and often does lead to chronic illness and disease.

Just like your house needs cleaning for the removal of dust and dirt, so does the body. The systems utilized to rid itself of these toxins and waste are the kidneys, liver, lungs, blood (circulatory system), colon, lymphatic system, and skin.

The human body is a many-splendored mechanism.

The liver. The detoxification process starts in the liver. The amazing liver weighs about 3 pounds and is the second largest organ in the body, second only to skin, and is the only one that can regenerate itself. While the liver detox process is a complicated one, it essentially does this in two phases. In Phase 1, the liver filters blood and works to either neutralize the chemical or toxin or convert it to an intermediate form for Phase 2. Phase 2 works to further break down artificial chemicals and toxins that can then be safely excreted from the body. When the liver cannot keep up with the influx of toxins, or Phase 2 is slower than Phase 1, toxins will start to accumulate in the body. If this happens, the liver tries to store the toxins, so they do not circulate in the blood and cause illness or disease. Most toxins are fat soluble, so the liver will shuttle toxins off to fat cells for safe storage. The body will then hold onto these fat cells so that the toxins will not release back into the bloodstream. Thus, a body that is toxic is a body holding on to fat cells.

Kidneys. Kidneys filter waste and toxins out of the blood. They are responsible for taking waste out of other fluids in the body as well. Because they filter fluids, they also balance them. As they are filtering, kidneys release hormones into the body that are responsible for regulating blood pressure as well as controlling and stimulating the number of red blood cells that are produced. The process naturally creates Vitamin D and hormones that affect the function of other organs in the body.

Lungs. There are sensors in your brain that know when you need more oxygen or less carbon dioxide in your blood and cause you to breathe harder. Your lungs do more than move oxygen in and carbon dioxide out of the body. They also act as filters. Mucus in your lungs catches and holds dust, germs, and other things that have entered the lungs.

Blood. Blood is a body fluid in humans that delivers nutrients and oxygen to the cells and transports metabolic waste products away from those same cells. The blood is then filtered by the kidneys.

Colon. The colon, also known as the large intestine or large bowel, absorbs water from digested food. Muscular contractions of the colon move the waste left over from this process to the rectum. A bowel movement expels the solidified waste from the body.

Lymphatic system. The lymphatic system is part of the immune system. It maintains fluid balance and plays a role in absorbing fats and fat-soluble nutrients.
The lymphatic or lymph system involves an extensive network of vessels that passes through almost all our tissues to allow for the movement of a fluid called lymph. Lymph circulates through the

body in a similar way to blood. There are about 600 lymph nodes in the body. These nodes swell in response to infection, due to a build-up of lymph fluid, bacteria, or other organisms and immune system cells.

Skin. The oil in the skin which keeps our skin soft, this is produced thru oil ducts and can be used as another elimination method for toxins that are fat soluble. Normally the liver processes these and turns them into water solubles and the kidneys flush them out. If your liver is congested the body will call upon the skin to do the duty. Thus acne, blackheads, pimples, boils usually appear when toxins have been forced from the liver and/or kidneys towards the next and largest elimination channel, the skin.

Detox Dance.
Our body's detox system is an exquisite orchestra of organs, cells, and molecules that work hand in hand to achieve one goal- keeping us clean and healthy. It achieves this by neutralizing and eliminating toxic substances, waste materials, harmful bacteria, viruses, and infections. All the systems mentioned, work together to perform this function. To recap:

- the liver is the primary detoxifying organ of the body. It filters the blood from all toxic substances and impurities coming from the digestive tract.
- the intestines flush away waste materials from the body, support the immune system, and deliver nutrients to the bloodstream.
- the lymphatic system flushes away toxic substances and waste materials through circulating lymph, a colorless fluid containing white blood cells, throughout the body.
- the respiratory system filters the air we breathe and provides fresh oxygen for the body, flush out carbon dioxide as well as other waste gases through exhalation.

- they kidneys filter out the wastes and toxins present in the fluids in the body.
- the skin provides cover and protection against the environment.
- the immune systems monitor all the parts of the body for foreign invaders and trigger the appropriate response accordingly.

Besides helping you eliminate the wrong foods that can contribute to weight gain, the right detox program can give your liver and overall health a helping hand eliminating those excess toxins.

Many detox for weight loss. The key is to detox for quality of life. When we cleanse our systems of the daily toxins that we breathe, eat, absorb, consume, our overall health improves, our mental health improves, our cravings for the foods that heal and help the body thrive, and the weight comes off naturally. The best thing about the change in lifestyle, is the changes are sustained. The weight comes off and stays off. The clarity of the skin improves and stays clear and glowing. The need for prescribed medicines diminishes and stays gone. When speaking about quality of life, we want sustained change!

Signs your body provides you that you are in toxin overload are brain fog, constipation, fatigue, weight gain, unfamiliar body odor, chemical sensitivities, physical discomfort, skin problems, and insomnia. This overload comes by way of the numerous products we use each day on our bodies and in our home, the foods we consume riddled with artificial chemicals from mass production, and the environment by way of pollutants in our environment from massive lifestyle changes. The industrial revolution greatly altered the general population living in balance with nature. Now with the population tipping critical mass, the earth is overloaded with pollution.

With this revelation, does this mean a total exodus of all artificial chemicals and all things "unnatural." For those who lack the proper education, the knee jerk answer is yes. However, chemicals are all around us. Essential oils, herbs, and all things found in both nature and the laboratory are or contain chemicals.

Thus, the answer is not necessarily total elimination. Moderation is typically what works and shows proven results for the majority. For some, total elimination works. There is no right way or wrong way—it is just a matter of knowing which strategy works better for you. There are those who have an all or nothing mindset and thus have no issue with ridding their routine of everything one considers "bad."

For many, this is an unrealistic goal doomed for failure before it even starts. Making small, deliberate changes that are achievable is how to make real change for these folks. If one has a habit of eating fast food each day for lunch, to expect a total annihilation of fast food from one's diet cold turkey has a low probability for success. On the other hand, if the first goal for the week is to cut back one meal and substitute with a healthy alternative, that is a highly achievable goal. This strategy also helps with managing the withdrawal symptoms. US researchers have found that junk food addicts who go cold turkey can experience everything from mood swings to cravings, anxiety, headaches, and poor sleep.

Fasting

Another method of detoxing or purging the toxins from the body is to fast. What is fasting? Fasting is the willful refrainment from eating and drinking. In a physiological context, fasting may refer to the metabolic status of a person who has not eaten overnight, or to the metabolic state achieved after complete digestion and absorption of a meal. Plainly, it is denial.

Why is it important? Fasting cleanses our body of toxins and forces cells into processes that are not usually stimulated when a steady stream of fuel from food is always present. When we fast, the body does not have its usual access to glucose, forcing the cells to resort to other means and materials to produce energy. As a result, the body begins gluconeogenesis, a natural process of producing its own sugar. The liver helps by converting non-carbohydrate materials like lactate, amino acids, and fats into glucose energy. Because our bodies conserve energy during fasting, our basal metabolic rate, or the amount of energy our bodies burn while resting, becomes more efficient, thereby lowering our heart rate and blood pressure. Fasting puts the body under mild stress, which makes our cells adapt by enhancing their ability to cope. In other words, they become strong.

There are several options in fasting. There is time-restricted feeding where one limits caloric intake to a specific timeframe. The vast majority undergo this when asleep. Then there is intermittent caloric restriction. This approach puts the body through short and intensive therapy. The intermittent calorie restriction approach also reminds us that we do not need to consume constantly. When we do consume, we can choose wisely and continue normal activities and exercise with reduced fuel. A third type of fasting is periodic fasting with diets that mimic fasting. The fasting mimicking plan essentially tricks your metabolism into thinking you are on a prolonged fast—while allowing you to eat. If you are fit and healthy, the fasting mimicking may be an option for you however should be done under the guidance of a registered dietitian or other health professional.

Exercise

Energy
If you eat healthy, small snacks and meals throughout the day, you will keep your blood sugar from crashing and feel more energetic. If you hit the gym for 30 minutes each day, you will have the added

benefit of a neurotransmitter called serotonin, which is a natural mood booster.

Weight Control
Losing weight and keeping it off takes a combination of eating fewer calories and burning more energy. Eat nutrient-dense, low-calorie foods such as fruits, vegetables and lean meats and other proteins that will fill you up. Integrate physical activity into your everyday routine in addition to scheduled exercise. For instance, take the stairs at work or park at the far end of the lot.

Health
Regular exercise and good nutrition may ameliorate or prevent a myriad of conditions including heart disease, hypertension, stroke, Type 2 diabetes, arthritis, osteoporosis, and depression. Consult your physician to make sure your diet and exercise plans are compatible with your medications and health conditions.

Improved Mental Well-Being
Built up toxins affect our mood. Toxic heavy metals are found in the air we breathe, the food we eat, and the houses we live in. These toxins accumulate, a phenomenon known as bioaccumulation, occurs as re-exposure happens before the body can rid itself of the previous exposure. This toxic metal exposure can result in a wide array of common mental health disorders that can mimic many psychiatric "diseases" and thus lead to psychoactive prescription drug use or other unnecessary treatments. Research shows that certain toxic substances have the potential to disrupt normal brain physiology and to impair neurological homeostasis. As well as headache, cognitive dysfunction, memory disturbance, and other neurological signs and symptoms, disruption of brain function may also manifest as subtle or overt alteration in thoughts, moods, or behaviors.

In the US, 1 in 10 adults suffers from depression. Three substances that have the greatest impact on human health are mercury, lead, and arsenic. Exposure to these toxic metals is known to cause anxiety and/or depression.

Fasting improves a host of metabolic functions. It lowers inflammation, improves blood pressure and lipids, and reduces inflammatory belly fat. Purging or cleansing the body of these toxins of crucial to mind body restoration, not to mention the restoration of wellbeing produces a reinvigoration of the spirit.

Sleep
Sleep is essential. It is the way the body heals itself. Without proper restoration of the mind and body, physical ailments can invade in body and the brain cannot function properly. This can impair your abilities to concentrate, think clearly, and process memories. For adults 18-60 years of age, The American Academy of Sleep Medicine and the Sleep Research Society recommends 7 or more hours sleep each night. The National Sleep Foundation recommends 7-9 hours for this same group. For most adults, at least seven hours of sleep each night is needed for proper cognitive and behavioral functions. Again, an insufficient amount of sleep can lead to serious repercussions. Some studies have shown sleep deprivation leaves people vulnerable to attention lapses, reduced cognition, delayed reactions, and mood shifts. Thus, getting adequate sleep is of critical important. The quality of this sleep is another issue.

Time in bed does not always equate to time spent sleeping. A way of gauging the quality of your sleep, ask yourself the following:
- Are you sleeping at least 85 percent of the total time in bed?
- Do you fall asleep in 30 minutes or less?
- Are you waking no more than once per night?
- When waking, do you remain awake for no more than 20 minutes before falling back asleep?

If you can answer yes to all of these, chances are those hours you are spending lying in bed are of quality.

If you answer no to one or more, here are some tips to possibly improve your sleep.

- Bedtime routines are key.
    - Take a relaxing bath.
    - Brush your teeth.
    - Wash your face.
    - Pray/Meditate.
    - Have sex.
- Be consistent. Go to bed at the same time each night and get up at the same time each morning, including on the weekends.
- Make sure your bedroom is quiet, dark, relaxing, and at a comfortable temperature.
- Remove electronic devices such as TVs, computers, and smart phones from the bedroom.
- Avoid large meals, caffeine, and alcohol before bedtime.
- Do not use tobacco.
- Exercise. Being physically active during the day can help you fall asleep more easily at night.

Chapter 19: The Bottom Line

Now or later? Either way you pay!

According to the American Medical Association (AMA), more than 75 percent of monies spent on healthcare today go toward treating people with chronic conditions such as high blood pressure, diabetes and heart disease. An unhealthy diet is one of the leading risk factors for poor health, accounting for up to 45% of all deaths from cardiometabolic diseases, such as heart disease, stroke, and type 2 diabetes.

Proper nutrition offers one of the most effective and least costly ways to decrease the burden of chronic and non-communicable diseases and their risk factors, including obesity. While a small percentage of our population will develop those diseases without high-risk lifestyle choices, it should be noted that it is becoming more prevalent due to factors such as obesity and a more sedentary lifestyle. In fact, the AMA reports that rates of obesity and diabetes have doubled over the past 25 years.

What are the causes and risk factors of obesity? The largest contributor, lifestyle which includes diet, exercise, sleep, and stress. This is a significant shift in recent times from genetics, the once prevailing determiner.   According to a National Center of Health Statistics 2003 survey, about 65.2 percent of American adults are overweight or obese as a result of poor nutrition. Obesity is defined as having a body mass index of 25 or more. Being overweight puts people at risk for developing a host of disorders and conditions, some of them life-threatening.

With lifestyle being the biggest contributor to lack of health in the US, the right interventions can reduce your risk. A healthy diet is one of the best ways to ward off these diseases. For example, the Mediterranean diet, high in vegetables, healthy fats, nuts, and fish, has been linked to a reduction in cardiovascular disease, but it is not the only one.

Know your numbers.

To lower your risk factors, you must lower your cholesterol. Keeping your cholesterol in check starts by knowing your numbers. If your cholesterol is borderline or high. It is time to act. Whether that includes making dietary changes, exercise, western medicine, or other medical interventions, acting is key.

Control your blood pressure. The American College of Cardiology and American Heart Association recently revamped their joint guidelines regarding blood pressure, essentially lowering the definition for high blood pressure to 130/80 from 140/90. What does this mean for you? If your blood pressure is under 140/90 but meets the new definition for high blood pressure, it does not necessarily mean you need to go on medication. What it does mean is that you should be even more vigilant about being physically active and making lifestyle modifications. It is a warning sign that you need to heed. There is a relationship between even moderate increases in blood pressure and increased risk of heart disease and stroke.

Weigh yourself.
The body mass index, or BMI, is a calculation used to determine your level of body fat. In some cases, it can help a doctor determine your overall fitness and your risk of developing chronic diseases. A normal BMI is between18.5 and 25; a person with a BMI between 25 and 30 is considered overweight; and a person with a BMI over 30 is considered obese. A person is considered underweight if the BMI is less than 18.5. According to a National Center of Health Statistics, results from the 2017-2018 National Health and Nutrition Examination Survey, about 30.7 percent of American adults are overweight, 42.4 percent are obese, and 9.2 percent are suffering from severe obesity. As with most measures of health, BMI is not a perfect test.

In general, the higher your BMI, the higher the risk of developing a range of conditions linked with excess weight, including:

- diabetes
- arthritis
- liver disease
- various types of cancer, i.e., breast, colon, and prostate
- high blood pressure or hypertension
- high cholesterol
- sleep apnea.

As a single measure, BMI is clearly not a perfect measure of health. It is still a useful starting point for important conditions that become more likely when a person is overweight or obese. Thus, it is a good idea to know your BMI.

Understanding the medical costs associated with poor nutrition is pertinent, as important as realizing the overall impact nutrition has on your total health. It can lead to behavioral health issues as proper nutrition and diet affect how you feel, look, think, and act. An unhealthy diet results in lower core strength, reduced focus, slower problem solving ability, and diminished muscle response time. Overall, malnutrition creates many negative health effects and result in an exponential increase in medical costs.

Closing

What to do with all this information? If nothing else, hopefully you are leaving this feeling more informed about the importance of reading food labels, increased confidence in interpreting these labels, and a heightened sense of the implications of not paying attention to what is in the food you and your family are eating.

It is a lot to take in and it is my hope you will re-read this book as many times as you need to reach your awareness goals. To recap, a couple great rules of thumb to take with you as you go forward in your grocery store adventures:

- find products with no more than five ingredients, and
- if you do not recognize or cannot pronounce the list of ingredients, LEAVE IT!

Thank you for trusting me enough to all me to accompany/guide you on your journey towards better health.   Remember, the key to a living a balanced life is ultimately…… Moderation!

Best wishes on your journey and thank you for allowing me to be a part of your narrative!